Curbside Consultation in Pediatric Sleep Disorders

49 Clinical Questions

Curbside Consultation in Pediatrics
Series

Series Editor, Lisa B. Zaoutis, MD

Curbside Consultation in Pediatric Sleep Disorders

49 Clinical Questions

EDITOR

Aaron S. Chidekel, MD
Associate Professor of Pediatrics
Sidney Kimmel Medical College at Thomas Jefferson University
Chief, Division of Pulmonology
Nemours/Alfred I. duPont Hospital for Children
Wilmington, Delaware

CRC Press
Taylor & Francis Group
Boca Raton London New York

CRC Press is an imprint of the
Taylor & Francis Group, an **informa** business

First published 2016 by SLACK Incorporated

Published 2024 by CRC Press
2385 NW Executive Center Drive, Suite 320, Boca Raton FL 33431

and by CRC Press
4 Park Square, Milton Park, Abingdon, Oxon, OX14 4RN

CRC Press is an imprint of Taylor & Francis Group, LLC

Library of Congress Cataloging-in-Publication Data

Curbside consultation in pediatric sleep disorders : 49 clinical questions / editor, Aaron S. Chidekel.
p. ; cm. -- (Curbside consultation in pediatrics series)
Pediatric sleep disorders Includes bibliographical references and index.
ISBN 978-1-61711-601-8 (alk. paper)
I. Chidekel, Aaron S., editor. II. Title: Pediatric sleep disorders. III. Series: Curbside consultation in pediatrics series.
[DNLM: 1. Child. 2. Infant. 3. Sleep Disorders--diagnosis. 4. Sleep Disorders--therapy. WL 108]
RJ506.S55
618.92'8498--dc23

2015029682

ISBN: 9781617116018 (pbk)
ISBN: 9781003523680 (ebk)

DOI: 10.1201/9781003523680

Dedication

For Stacy and the other three "C's."
For my parents, who first instilled in me a love of books.

Contents

Acknowledgments

I thank and acknowledge all of my colleagues, who continue to challenge me with important questions, and the patients, who trust me and rely on me to find answers. Particular thanks to my friend and colleague, Kate Cronan, MD, for her thoughtful and thorough review of the manuscript and to Carl Gartner, MD, who got me back into sleep medicine at the duPont Hospital for Children.

About the Editor

Aaron S. Chidekel, MD received his medical degree from Brown University in Providence, Rhode Island. He completed his internship and residency in general pediatrics at Yale-New Haven Hospital in Connecticut. He completed fellowship training in pediatric respiratory medicine in the Section of Pediatric Respiratory Medicine at Yale University School of Medicine. After completing this training, Dr. Chidekel moved to Nemours at the Alfred I. duPont Hospital for Children in Wilmington, Delaware, where he is currently the Chief of the Division of Pulmonology and Sleep Medicine. He directs a busy, accredited pediatric sleep medicine program at the Alfred I. duPont Hospital for Children. Dr. Chidekel is an Associate Professor of Pediatrics at the Sidney Kimmel Medical College of Thomas Jefferson University in Philadelphia, Pennsylvania. He has authored numerous scientific papers and abstracts regarding various aspects of clinical and basic research related to pediatric pulmonary medicine. He has edited and contributed chapters to several textbooks and has served as a reviewer for many prestigious journals as well. He is a fellow in the American Academy of Pediatrics and has been active as an officer and board member of the Delaware Chapter, and he is a member of the American Thoracic Society and the American Academy of Sleep Medicine.

Contributing Authors

Louella Amos, MD (Questions 27, 29)
Department of Pediatrics
Division of Pulmonary and Sleep Medicine
Children's Hospital of Wisconsin
Milwaukee, Wisconsin

Kari Baber, PhD (Question 19)
Children's Hospital of Philadelphia
Philadelphia, Pennsylvania

Suzanne E. Beck, MD (Question 28)
Medical Director, Sleep Laboratory
Children's Hospital of Philadelphia
Philadelphia, Pennsylvania

Anita Bhandari, MD (Question 37)
Division of Pediatric Pulmonology
Department of Pediatrics
University of Connecticut School of Medicine
Farmington, Connecticut
Connecticut Children's Medical Center
Hartford, Connecticut

Michael Blechner, MD (Question 37)
Department of Pediatrics
University of Connecticut School of Medicine
Farmington, Connecticut
Division of Pediatric Pulmonology,
Connecticut Children's Medical Center
Hartford, Connecticut

Todd Burchard, BS, RPSGT, RST (Questions 47, 49)
Lead Polysomnographic Technologist
Sleep Medicine Program
Division of Pulmonology
Nemours/Alfred I. duPont Hospital for Children
Wilmington, Delaware

Christina Calamaro, PhD, CRNP (Question 20)
Director of Research and Innovation for Patient Services
Nemours/Alfred I. duPont Hospital for Children
Wilmington, Delaware

Johanna Carpenter, PhD (Question 19)
Nemours/Alfred I. duPont Hospital for Children
Wilmington, Delaware

Mohammad Cheema, MD (Question 8)
Pediatric Sleep Center of New Orleans
Kenner, Louisiana

Jennifer L. Curran, PhD (Question 17)
Licensed Psychologist
Eastern Maine Medical Center
Developmental Pediatrics
Bangor, Maine

Lynn A. D'Andrea, MD (Questions 27, 29, 34)
Professor of Pediatrics
Chief, Division of Pulmonary and Sleep Medicine
Medical College of Wisconsin
Children's Hospital of Wisconsin
Milwaukee, Wisconsin

Ritu Grewal, MD (Questions 4, 23)
Assistant Professor of Medicine
Attending Physician, Sleep Disorders Center
Attending Physician, Division of Pulmonary Medicine
Thomas Jefferson University Hospital
Philadelphia, Pennsylvania

Robert Heinle, MD (Questions 7, 15, 16)
Pulmonary Division
Nemours/Alfred I. duPont Hospital for Children
Wilmington, Delaware

Cheyenne Hughes-Reid, PhD (Question 18)
Pediatric Psychologist
Nemours/Alfred I. duPont Hospital for Children
Wilmington, Delaware
Assistant Professor of Pediatrics
Jefferson Medical College
Philadelphia, Pennsylvania

Persephone Jones, MD, MPH (Question 14)
Chief, Division of Developmental Medicine
Nemours/Alfred I. duPont Hospital
for Children
Wilmington, Delaware

Lewis J. Kass, MD (Questions 31, 45)
Westchester Pediatric Pulmonology and
Sleep Medicine
Mount Kisco, New York

Holger Link, MD (Questions 21, 22, 30)
Clinical Associate Professor
Department of Pediatrics
Oregon Health & Science University
Portland, Oregon

Floyd Livingston, MD (Questions 3, 5, 6)
NCCO Cystic Fibrosis Foundation Center
Medical Director
Division Chief, Pediatric Pulmonology
Nemours Children's Clinic-Orlando
Associate Professor of Pediatrics
The Florida State University School of
Medicine
Assistant Professor of Pediatrics
University of Central Florida College
of Medicine
Nemours Children's Clinic-Orlando
Orlando, Florida

Jennifer L. Maher, DO (Question 9)
Fellow, Neonatal-Perinatal Medicine
Thomas Jefferson University
Philadelphia, Pennsylvania

Jennifer A. Marriner, MSN, CPNP (Questions 11, 46)
Department of Pulmonology/Sleep Medicine
Nemours/Alfred I. duPont Hospital
for Children
Wilmington, Delaware

Meghan McAuliffe Lines, PhD (*Question 18*)
Co-Director of Behavioral Health
Chief Psychologist
Nemours/Alfred I. duPont Hospital
for Children
Wilmington, Delaware

Raj Padman, MD (*Question 32*)
Division of Pulmonology and Sleep Medicine
Nemours/Alfred I. duPont Hospital
for Children
Wilmington, Delaware

Vandna Passi, MD (*Questions 35, 36*)
Nemours/Alfred I. duPont Hospital
for Children
Wilmington, Delaware

David A. Paul, MD (*Questions 9, 13*)
Associate Director of Neonatology
Christiana Care Health System
Newark, Delaware
Professor of Pediatrics
Jefferson Medical College
Philadelphia, Pennsylvania

Amy Renwick, MD (*Question 12*)
Nemours/Alfred I. duPont Hospital
for Children
Wilmington, Delaware

Marianne C. San Antonio, DO (*Question 39*)
Nemours/Alfred I. duPont Hospital
for Children
Wilmington, Delaware

Vanessa Shanks, MD (*Question 13*)
Fellow, Neonatal-Perinatal Medicine
Thomas Jefferson University
Philadelphia, Pennsylvania

Ambika Shenoy, MD (*Question 38*)
Division of Pulmonology and Sleep Medicine
Nemours/Alfred I. duPont Hospital
for Children
Wilmington, Delaware

Jennifer Shroff Pendley, PhD (*Questions 17, 40*)
Co-Director of Behavioral Health
Chief Psychologist
Nemours/Alfred I. duPont Hospital
for Children
Wilmington, Delaware

Gabor Szuhay, MD (*Questions 24, 25, 26*)
Pediatric Neurologist and Diplomate of Sleep Medicine
Assistant Professor at University of Illinois
Consultant Pediatric Neurologist at Children's Hospital of Illinois
Geisinger Medical Center, Pennsylvania
Women's and Children's Hospital of
Huntsville, Alabama

Ignacio E. Tapia, MD (*Question 33*)
Attending Physician, Sleep Center
Division of Pulmonary Medicine
The Children's Hospital of Philadelphia
Philadelphia, Pennsylvania

Rhonda Walter, MD (*Questions 14, 39*)
Division of Developmental Medicine
Nemours/Alfred I duPont Hospital for Children
Wilmington, Delaware

Rocio Zeballos-Chavez, MD (*Question 34*)
Sleep Fellow
Medical College of Wisconsin
Children's Hospital of Wisconsin
Milwaukee, Wisconsin

Foreword

While the importance of a good night's sleep to the development and optimal functioning of a child of any age is undisputed, pediatric sleep medicine is a relatively new area of scientific inquiry and clinical medicine. As such, few user-friendly, concise, and practical references are available to the primary care provider. *Curbside Consultation in Pediatric Sleep Medicine: 49 Clinical Questions* is just this resource. This book is targeted to the busy practitioner who requires a ready reference when he or she has a sleep-related question or concern about a patient in the office, whether it is related to a normal variant of sleep, a behavioral sleep problem, or possible sleep-disordered breathing. This book will provide the reader with an introduction to this broad and important area of pediatric medical practice.

Curbside Consultation in Pediatric Sleep Medicine: 49 Clinical Questions provides the busy clinician with a thorough, yet concise, overview of the various aspects of pediatric sleep medicine. Covering topics ranging from the basic nuts and bolts of sleep and its development throughout infancy and childhood to the complexities of polysomnography, the reader will become familiar with how to approach a child with a potential sleep disorder. The various and common types of respiratory and nonrespiratory sleep disorders are covered, along with chapters on the unique aspects of sleep and breathing in infants and in children with underlying genetic, medical, and neuropsychiatric conditions. Behavioral sleep problems and normal variants of sleep are detailed as well. Finally, important and challenging topics, such as the diagnosis and management of sleep problems and sleep deprivation in adolescents, are also covered in detail in the book.

Pediatric sleep medicine is a broad and wide-ranging subject. To provide clinical insight into its many varied conditions and manifestations, *Curbside Consultation in Pediatric Sleep Medicine: 49 Clinical Questions* collects the expertise of a diverse group of experts in the field into one easy-to-use reference. Representing a variety of backgrounds, including pulmonology, developmental medicine, neonatology, psychology, and neurology, as well as nursing and sleep technology, all of these highly qualified contributors share their clinical expertise while reviewing some of the latest literature in the field. All of the contributors to the book are themselves busy clinicians, seeing the same patients and facing the same challenges as their colleagues in general medical practice. They truly are the experts who should be providing practical, succinct advice and answers to the challenging clinical questions of their peers and colleagues.

Sleep is a universal necessity and sleep disorders are a common pediatric problem. I am convinced that the busy, pediatric practitioner, and even the trainee, will find this book to be an invaluable introduction and resource in his or her daily practices. The questions asked in its chapters are practical and pertinent, and the answers provided are relevant, patient-focused, and valuable to the patients and families for whom we provide care.

Carl Gartner, MD
Professor of Pediatrics
Vice-Chairman of Pediatrics, Emeritus
Sidney Kimmel Medical College at Thomas Jefferson University
Director of Pediatrics, Emeritus
Nemours/Alfred I. duPont Hospital for Children

Introduction

Pediatric sleep medicine is a relatively new pediatric subspecialty. It is a broad and important topic that spans many areas of medical practice and is as relevant to neonates and infants as it is to older children and adolescents. Pediatric sleep medicine is a diverse and multidisciplinary area as well. Covering an array of topics and involving varied practitioners ranging from neonatology to neurology and pulmonology to psychiatry and psychology, pediatric sleep medicine has something of interest to challenge every one of us caring for children. Indeed, since all children sleep, all of us who provide care to them will potentially be involved in evaluating, treating, and, hopefully, solving children's sleep problems.

Pediatric sleep medicine is a diverse subject, and trying to prioritize subjects for this book was challenging. In selecting the most pertinent topics for questions in *Curbside Consultation in Pediatric Sleep Medicine: 49 Clinical Questions*, this diversity of subject matter and practitioners was celebrated. Every effort was made to include a wide array of topics so that the spectrum of sleep medicine and sleep disorders would be reflected and represented. From behavioral sleep problems to sleep-disordered breathing and a myriad of other topics, this book is specifically designed to provide a quick introduction to many of the common and key issues in pediatric sleep medicine.

Curbside Consultation in Pediatric Sleep Medicine: 49 Clinical Questions is designed to be a useful resource for the student just learning about pediatric sleep medicine or the seasoned practitioner in need of a quick clinical reference, or even a refresher, on this broad and important area of pediatric practice. I hope you enjoy it and would not hesitate to stop me in the hallway again for another curbside consult on this or any other clinical topic that is puzzling you.

SECTION I

THE ABCs OF SLEEP

QUESTION 1

Why Do We Sleep and What Is Happening When Children Sleep?

Aaron S. Chidekel, MD

The precise purpose of sleep remains unclear, but it is certainly a necessity. If one stays awake too long, the intrinsic drive to sleep will overcome any conscious desire for wakefulness. If experimental animals are deprived of sleep long enough, death ensues. Sleep is also clearly a requirement for the optimal physical, emotional, social, and cognitive functioning of a child. Indeed, learning and behavior are impacted by sleep deprivation or sleep fragmentation. A child's sleep pattern is also critical to the optimal functioning of a family and it is a source of great stress and distress when a child's sleep difficulties impact the rhythms of family life. Unfortunately, the sleep-wake cycle of a child and his or her family is often very out of balance before a practitioner becomes aware of any concern and, much to the dismay of both the parent and the practitioner, a rapid solution is often out of the question by this time.

During infancy, eye closure is the most reliable sign of sleep, and wakeful behaviors such as suckling, whimpering, or even crying may persist in the initial moments of normal infant sleep. However, with age and central nervous system development, the more familiar mature patterns of sleep become apparent. The body is still and peaceful and, indeed, frequent or unusual movements during sleep may be the sign of an underlying sleep disorder. Similarly, breathing during sleep should also be quiet and peaceful. Snoring, gasping, or irregular breathing may also be a sign of underlying sleep disorder. Breathing during sleep in a healthy child should be a subtle finding. Sleep is often further described as a state of reversible disengagement from the environment associated with relaxed posture and muscle tone and reduced, but not absent, responsiveness to environmental input and stimuli. While most often appearing quiescent externally, sleep is a time of intense neural activity as the brain cycles though the stages of rapid eye movement (REM) and NREM sleep. Other bodily systems and functions undergo important transitions during sleep as well, as will be briefly outlined next.

Over the years, many theories about the purpose of sleep have been proposed. These include a central role for sleep in energy conservation, self preservation and species adaptation, physical restoration, developmental facilitation, and learning and memory processing. Each of these theories has its own basis in physiological or anthropological evidence, but none has been proved with

Chidekel AS, ed. *Curbside Consultation in Pediatric Sleep Disorders: 49 Clinical Questions* (pp. 3-5)

certainty. For example, although it is true that less energy is expended by the body during sleep, the amount of energy conserved is quite minimal for the time spent sleeping. Moreover, brain activity and energy usage during REM sleep are actually quite similar to when one is awake. In fact, REM sleep has been described as a wakeful brain in a paralyzed body. The notion of sleep-related physical restoration is centered on the conservation of deep stage 3 (slow wave sleep)—meaning that, after a period of sleep deprivation, slow wave sleep is replenished first. A number of important endocrine and immune functions are also linked to this stage of sleep, such as the secretion of growth hormone, which may provide additional credence to this theory of sleep. Currently, however, the focus of much of the research on the true purpose of sleep centers on brain development, learning, and memory processing. Sleep in general, but particularly REM sleep, seems to be an important time for the pruning and facilitation of synapses and neural networks throughout the brain, and these functions are thought to be critical for learning, memory processing, and the facilitation (or pruning back) of synaptic connections.

Sleep is, thus, anything but a passive state. It has a specific organization that evolves strikingly with the development and the eventual aging of a person over his or her lifetime (as will be discussed further in Question 8). Organized into cycles of non-REM (NREM) and REM sleep, the brain and body cycle through each of these sleep states several times during the main sleep period. Each sleep stage is defined by specific electroencephalographic (EEG), electrooculographic (EOG), and electromyographic (EMG) features (these will be described in detail in Question 3). After infancy, sleep is entered into through light, NREM sleep and, at the moment of sleep onset, a person becomes unaware of his or her surroundings and short-term memory function ceases. Stage 1 NREM sleep is a transitional period and stage 2 sleep soon follows. Deep, slow wave stage 3 sleep occurs thereafter and, as discussed previously, it is this deepest stage of sleep—when a person is least arousable and aware of their surroundings—that is highly protected and conserved. REM, or dream sleep, completes the sleep cycle, which can be as short as 45 minutes in an infant and as long as 90 minutes in an older child or adult. In infancy, REM sleep is much more predominant than in older children and adults. In early childhood, deep stage 3 sleep is the most prevalent stage of sleep, which then falls off toward adolescence and adulthood.

Bodily functions are also greatly altered during sleep compared to wakefulness. During sleep, and especially during NREM sleep, parasympathetic tone is predominant. There is relatively increased sympathetic tone during REM sleep. The predominance of parasympathetic tone leads to many of the physical characteristics that can be recognized during NREM sleep (namely, regular respirations and heart rate); however, during REM sleep, bursts of respiratory, heart rate, and blood pressure variability can be recognized observationally and correspond with spikes in sympathetic nervous system output. Respiratory function during sleep is discussed in detail in Question 4. Temperature regulation is also altered during the different stages of sleep. Body temperature follows a 24-hour circadian rhythm that results in slight variations in core temperature during the circadian cycle. In general, body temperature rises during the circadian day and begins to fall off during the circadian night, reaching a nadir in the early hours of the morning, ideally when a person is sleeping. Body temperature falls independently during sleep compared to wakefulness, particularly during NREM sleep, and this is likely due in part to decreased energy consumption. Interestingly, temperature regulation is absent during REM sleep and mechanisms such as perspiration and shivering are absent. Endocrine function changes during sleep as well. A number of hormonal systems are linked to sleep and the circadian timing system. The most notable examples of these include growth hormone secretion, which is closely linked to deep stage 3 sleep; thyroid stimulating hormone, which is suppressed by sleep; and, finally, cortisol secretion, which rises prior to wake time and decreases in the evening prior to sleep. Melatonin, a hormone for which secretion is also closely linked to the circadian rhythm, will be discussed in Question 44. Finally, a number of other systems change their levels of activity during sleep. For example, gastrointestinal motility and urine production both decrease during sleep, with obvious advantages. Primary nocturnal enuresis is a common occurrence in young children, due in part to their smaller bladders and higher proportion of deep sleep. However, secondary enuresis may be associated with such sleep disorders as obstructive sleep apnea syndrome, among its many other clinical considerations.

Summary

Although much about the purpose of sleep remains a mystery, its critical role in the health and well being of a person is crystal clear. Far from being a passive state, sleep is an active and well-organized process that is both required and highly conserved. Many important bodily functions are altered during sleep, and still others follow a circadian regularity that is complemented by sleep. When sleep is deprived, disrupted, or abnormal because of an underlying sleep or nervous system disorder, optimal learning, development, and overall functioning are adversely affected. Indeed, normal sleep is critical to the social, emotional, physical, and cognitive development and functioning of each of us and, therefore, the recognition of sleep difficulties and disorders in childhood is central to pediatric practice.

Suggested Readings

Jenni OG, LeBourgeois MK. Understanding sleep-wake behavior and sleep disorders in children: the value of a model. *Curr Opin Psychiatry.* 2006;19(3):282-287.

Markov D, Goldman M. Normal sleep and circadian rhythms: neurobiological mechanisms underlying sleep and wakefulness. *Psychiatr Clin N Am.* 2006;29:841-853.

Sheldon SH. The function, phylogeny and ontogeny of sleep. In: Sheldon SH, Ferber R, Kryger MR, Gozal D, eds. *Principles and Practice of Pediatric Sleep Medicine.* 2nd ed. Philadelphia: Elsevier Saunders; 2014:3-11.

Silber MH. Staging sleep. *Sleep Medicine Clinics.* 2009;4:343-352.

Sleep: What It Is—How It Works—Why We Do It—What Can Go Wrong. Available at: http://howsleepworks.com/index.html. Accessed March 10, 2015.

QUESTION 2

What Are the Nuts and Bolts of Sleep and Its Regulation?

Aaron S. Chidekel, MD

The neurophysiologic basis of sleep is rooted in the function of specific brain structures and neurotransmitter systems that mediate and modulate wakefulness and sleep in a synchronized fashion. Indeed, it is the interaction among these neural systems and structures that underlie the specific features of rapid eye movement (REM) and non-REM sleep. In addition to these complex neurophysiologic mechanisms, a simpler and more intuitive 2-process model of sleep-wake regulation composed of the intrinsic sleep drive (Process S) and an opposing circadian alerting system (Process C) is also a useful construct to consider when approaching a patient with a potential sleep disorder. A basic familiarity with these neural mechanisms, coupled with an understanding of the importance of a smooth and regular sleep-wake cycle, governed by the 2-process model, should provide a robust understanding of how sleep is regulated during the 24-hour day.

A full discussion of the neurophysiologic basis of sleep, which is complex, is beyond the scope of this chapter. However, a brief understanding of both the neuroanatomic basis of sleep and the main neurotransmitter systems involved in the promotion of sleep and wakefulness is both useful and clinically relevant. This is particularly the case when considering the potential influence of underlying neurological conditions, such as attention deficit hyperactivity disorder or epilepsy; the impact of supplements, such as melatonin; the effect of drugs, such as caffeine and alcohol; and the role of medications, such as anti-histamines and stimulants, on modulating sedation and arousal and the sleep-wake cycle. Similarly, environmental cues, such as light, temperature, and physical activity, can influence these neural systems as well, and also serve as important clues and adjuncts in the diagnosis and management of pediatric sleep disorders.

In the brain, there is not a single "sleep substance" or "sleep center" per se; rather, it is most useful to think of the brain as having wake-promoting, or alerting, areas and neurotransmitter systems as well as sleep-promoting, or inhibitory, areas and neurotransmitter systems. The coordinated and cyclical activity of these regions and neurotransmitter systems in the brain is critical to the onset and offset of sleep, as well as to the brain's cycling through the different stages of REM and non-REM sleep. Sleep onset and offset has a distinct neurophysiologic fingerprint as

Chidekel AS, ed. *Curbside Consultation in Pediatric Sleep Disorders: 49 Clinical Questions* (pp. 7-10)

does each stage of sleep, characterized by the synchronized function and inhibition of specific regions of the brain and specific neurotransmitter systems. These systems tend to be anatomically divergent and redundant and, similarly, there are a number of neurotransmitters that are primarily wake-promoting and neurotransmitters that are primarily sleep-promoting. Neurotransmitters important in the promotion of sleep include adenosine and gamma aminobutyric acid (GABA). Neurotransmitters important in the promotion of wakefulness include acetylcholine, dopamine, histamine, hypocretin/orexin, norepinephrine, and serotonin. Some neurotransmitters can have a dual function, depending on where a specific neuron is projecting. It is apparent that the facilitation or inhibition of these neurotransmitter systems will have profound effects on sleep and wakefulness. One of the structures in the brain that is particularly central to the regulation of sleep is the hypothalamus. The anterior hypothalamus is where the bilateral suprachiasmatic nuclei, the intrinsic biological clock and circadian timing mechanism, are located. The ventrolateral preoptic nucleus of the anterior hypothalamus contains important inhibitory neurons that secrete GABA, and which are important in inhibiting wake promoting areas of the brain. Finally, the posterior hypothalamus, and particularly the tuberomammillary nucleus, is an area of significant histaminergic and hypocretinergic input, which activates this group of neurons, resulting in the promotion of wakefulness. These hypothalamic structures are critical to the generation of non-REM sleep. REM sleep, on the other hand, is thought to be generated by complex neural interactions in the pons. In the pons, specific groups of "REM-on" and "REM-off" neurons project to other areas of the brain and spinal cord to promote or inhibit the conditions of an active brain in a paralyzed body that uniquely characterize REM sleep.

The 2-process model of sleep and wakefulness is a useful and practical construct to consider when approaching the timing and regulation of sleep and wakefulness. It is intuitive and does not require a thorough understanding of neuroanatomy and neurotransmitter systems. The 2-process model consists of a homeostatic mechanism (Process S), which is primarily sleep-promoting, and a circadian timing system (Process C), which is primarily wake-promoting. The homeostatic mechanism can be thought of as an intrinsic drive to sleep, which is based primarily on the duration and quality of the previous sleep period, and the duration of the current period of wakefulness. The longer one has been awake, the greater the pressure will be to sleep; and, with the occurrence of sleep, the pressure to sleep is dissipated, preparing the individual for the next period of wakefulness. If a person is sleep-deprived or if sleep is abnormal, the pressure to sleep will remain high and excessive daytime sleepiness will result. If a person is aroused by an environmental stimulus (eg, a sound in the night) and has insufficient intrinsic pressure to return to sleep, a prolonged nighttime awakening can result.

In the central nervous system, Process S is thought to be mediated by the accumulation of adenosine, which is a metabolite of brain functioning. Adenosine is also a neurotransmitter and neuromodulator that directly inhibits brain functions associated with wakefulness. As adenosine builds up in the brain, these wake-promoting processes are inhibited, the pressure to sleep is increased, and a person will begin to feel sleepy. This pressure to sleep increases until it becomes insurmountable and sleep occurs, whether planned for or not—such as when a sleepy toddler falls to sleep in the middle of a noisy room or a sleep-deprived teen nods off in class. This allows the adenosine to be cleared, thereby resetting the sleep "homeostat" and setting up the condition for the next period of wakefulness. As Process S is mediated by adenosine, it is also clear why caffeine, an adenosine antagonist, is such a potent promoter of wakefulness or insomnia. Taken in excess or at the wrong time of day, caffeine, through its inhibition of adenosine, will directly promote wakefulness.

Balanced against the primarily sleep-promoting homeostatic mechanism is the circadian timing system. The circadian timing system (Process C) is primarily wake-promoting. The circadian rhythm will be discussed in detail in Question 5. Briefly, the circadian system is the intrinsic biological clock, which resides in the hypothalamus and serves as the main mechanism that controls the timing of sleep and many other biological functions. The circadian system consists of a group of neurons with an intrinsic oscillation that approximates the 24-hour day. On average, it is slightly longer than 24 hours, but genetic factors result in some variation in this periodicity. Since the circadian system is not perfectly aligned with the 24-hour day, it must be set or synchronized with the world outside. Light is the strongest factor that can influence circadian timing, and exposure to light at an inopportune time can result in a shift in the circadian clock that can impact the timing and duration of sleep. For example, the lengthening of days with the coming of spring can make it difficult for a toddler to maintain an early bedtime because it is light outside, and, similarly, morning darkness can make it even more difficult for a sleepy adolescent to awaken in time for the school bus. Other important external circadian timing signals include the timing of meals and exercise, as well as ambient temperature.

Together, Process S, the sleep drive, and Process C, the circadian alerting system, should function in a well-coordinated fashion to regulate the timing and duration of sleep. When one awakens in the morning, the pressure to sleep should be minimal as long as the timing and duration of the previous sleep period was physiologic and sufficient. Throughout the day, as sleep pressure (Process S) slowly builds, it is opposed by the circadian timing system (Process C) so that an individual remains awake and alert (one important exception to this general rule is the well-recognized circadian lull that occurs in the afternoon). When night falls, however, the circadian timing system begins to slacken, primarily in response to the fall off in ambient light, which results in the secretion of melatonin from the pineal gland, thereby sending the biological signal that the time of main sleep period has arrived. Melatonin (see Question 44) is secreted throughout the main sleep period, in part to promote sleep maintenance as sleep pressure (Process S) is dissipated. In the second half of the sleep period, melatonin production is reduced, cortisol secretion increases, and the conditions for alertness are again favored—namely, the reduction in Process S and the resurgence of the circadian alerting system with the drop off in melatonin production and the return of the light of the day.

When the neural mechanisms that underlie sleep onset and offset are synchronized with the circadian and homeostatic systems, a child will cycle easily from wakefulness to sleep in a smooth and regular fashion and awaken refreshed, and learning, development, and daytime function will be optimized. However, when one component of this system is out of balance or impacted by a medical or environmental stressor, sleep disorders can result. For example, in narcolepsy (see Question 23), the neural mechanisms involving the hypocretin/orexin system in the hypothalamus are deficient, resulting in excessive sleepiness, sleep attacks, and abnormal regulation of REM sleep. When there is a mismatch between the circadian timing system and the sleep needs of an individual or an important social demand (eg, an early school start time), a circadian rhythm sleep disorder, such as delayed sleep phase syndrome, results (see Question 19). Finally, when the architecture of sleep itself is abnormal, or if sleep is disrupted and fragmented, as occurs in obstructive sleep apnea syndrome (see Question 27), the homeostatic mechanism cannot be reset and the child will have impaired daytime functioning due to excessive daytime sleepiness. To complicate matters further, these underlying mechanisms of sleep disorders can coexist and overlap, adding to the challenge of treating and counseling a parent about his or her child's sleep or treating childhood sleep disorders.

Suggested Readings

Borbély AA. A two process model of sleep regulation. *Hum Neurobiol.* 1982;1(3):195-204.

Daan S, Beersma DG, Borbély AA. Timing of human sleep: recovery process gated by a circadian pacemaker. *Am J Physiol.* 1984;246(2 Pt 2):R161-183.

Jenni OG, LeBourgeois MK. Understanding sleep-wake behavior and sleep disorders in children: the value of a model. *Curr Opin Psychiatry.* 2006;19(3):282-287.

Markov D, Goldman M. Normal sleep and circadian rhythms: neurobiological mechanisms underlying sleep and wakefulness. *Psychiatr Clin N Am.* 2006;29:841-853.

Saper CB, Scammell TE, Lu J. Hypothalamic regulation of sleep and circadian rhythms. *Nature.* 2005;437(7063): 1257-1263.

Siegel JM. The neurotransmitters of sleep. *J Clin Psychiatry.* 2004;65(S16):4-7.

QUESTION 3

What Are the Different Stages of Sleep?

Floyd Livingston, MD

Each sleep stage can be defined and characterized by evaluating its specific electroencephalographic (EEG), electrooculographic, and electromyographic features. Although the amounts and proportions of the different sleep stages evolve with human development over the lifetime of an individual, the characteristics of each sleep stage remain constant. By evaluating the different sleep stages, sleep quality and quantity can be defined, and the impact of development, sleep disorders, medications, and other factors on the sleep of an individual can be described.

During infancy, sleep is classified as active, quiet, or indeterminate. The infant brain has not yet fully developed to allow for full differentiation of the various sleep stages. Usually eye closure is the most reliable indicator of newborn or infant sleep. Infants have rapid sleep-to-wake transitions and the persistence of wakeful behaviors is seen; for example, sucking and swallowing activities often continue after an infant has fallen asleep. By the end of infancy, these rapid transitions smooth out to a pattern of more gradual transitions to sleep, accompanied by the state of drowsiness, and the evolution of more mature sleep cycling. Sleep cycles are 45 to 60 minutes at birth, but lengthen to approximately 90 minutes by 5 years of age. Dream or rapid eye movement (REM) sleep will occupy 50% of newborn sleep, but will gradually reduce to 20% to 25% of sleep time by 3 years of age. Similarly, in infancy, sleep onset REM sleep may be seen, whereas, in older children and adults, it is abnormal. Childhood sleep matures to adult patterns by late school age. The full EEG differentiation of slow wave and non-REM (NREM) sleep, along with the development of the adult patterns of sleep cycling and REM sleep, is also completed by the late school years.

During sleep onset and NREM sleep, responsiveness to external stimuli gradually decreases. At sleep onset, the individual becomes dissociated from his or her environment with loss of short-term memory, as well as decreased, and eventually absent, responses to mild auditory and visual stimuli. This altered perception of the environment is associated with altered neurotransmission at the level of the thalamus. The rhythmic, inhibitory oscillations generated by thalamus produce large, slow (delta) EEG waves that gradually "shut off" the excitatory neurons of the cortex. NREM sleep is divided into 3 stages. NREM sleep starts with drowsiness and progresses to very deep sleep, each defined by a unique EEG pattern. The alpha waves seen during quiet wakefulness

Chidekel AS, ed. *Curbside Consultation in Pediatric Sleep Disorders: 49 Clinical Questions* (pp. 11-14)

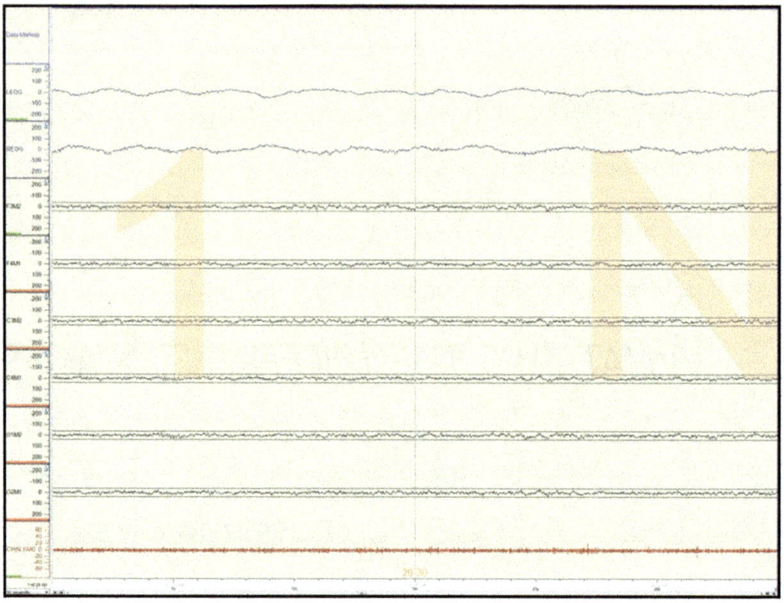

Figure 3-1. Stage I NREM sleep is characterized by low-voltage mixed-frequency EEG pattern, slow rolling eye movements, and low chin muscle tone.

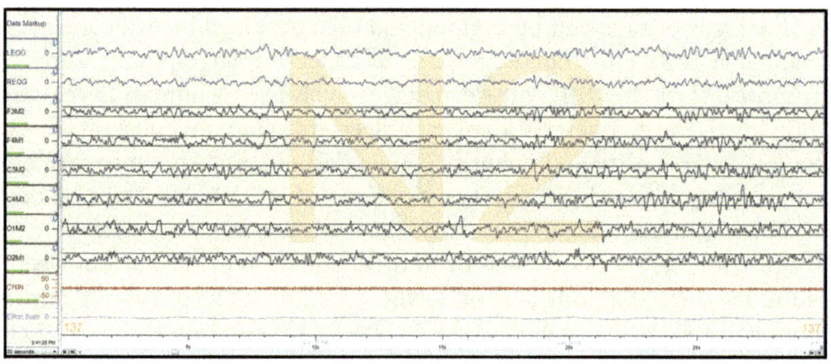

Figure 3-2. Stage II NREM sleep is characterized by specific EEG features, notably sleep spindles and K-complexes, absent eye movements, and low chin muscle tone.

are replaced by the slower theta waves. Stage I NREM sleep is a state of drowsiness and initial slowing of EEG pattern (Figure 3-1). A child can be easily and quickly aroused from initial sleep such as the classroom nod. Stage II sleep is defined by "sleep spindles" and "K-complexes" on the EEG (Figure 3-2). Arousal can still occur, although the waking will be longer and more confusing for the child. Stage III sleep is the deepest sleep for humans and has the very slowest and largest waves, delta waves (Figure 3-3). Arousal is very difficult during this stage. If arousal occurs during this stage, the child may be confused and disoriented. This arousal transition from sleeping to being awake during Stage III is quite difficult, and common NREM parasomnias—such as night terrors and sleepwalking—are seen during Stage III NREM sleep in the affected child.

During REM sleep, the EEG pattern is characterized by the appearance of low amplitude, mixed-frequency activity-desynchronized or activated pattern (Figure 3-4). Nerve impulses generated in the brain are transmitted to the spinal cord, but are blocked to prevent the acting out of dreams. All skeletal muscles are quiescent during REM sleep except for the respiratory, eye, and middle ear muscles. A child might appear paralyzed during REM sleep aside from an intermittent muscle twitch and the rapid eye twitching that the term *REM* denotes. Although muscle tone declines, both the heart rate and breathing patterns are essentially maintained. More oxygen is

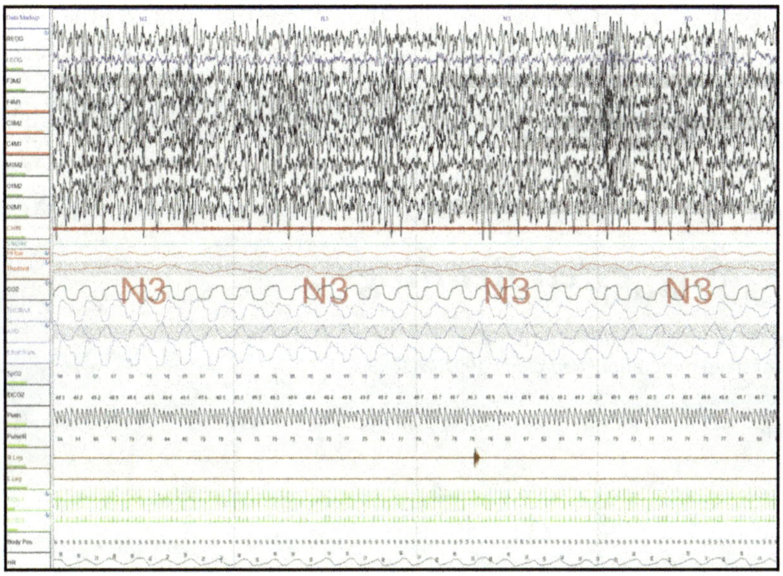

Figure 3-3. Stage III NREM sleep is characterized by large amplitude, low-frequency delta waves, absent eye movements, and low chin muscle tone. It is also characterized by slow and regular respirations and little cardiac variability.

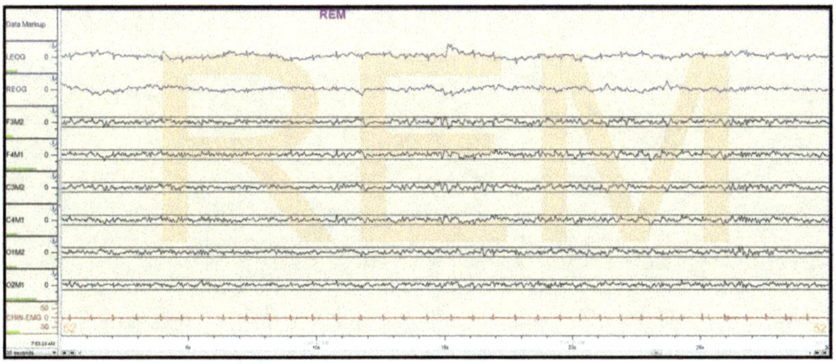

Figure 3-4. REM sleep is characterized by low-voltage mixed-frequency EEG pattern, the presence of rapid (sharp) eye movements, and absent chin muscle tone.

consumed and blood flow to the brain is increased during the dream state. EEG patterns become irregular, although rapid eye movements occur at a constant rate. The eyes are said to reflect the action of the dreams. REM dreaming is thought to serve to plant recent experiences into the brain's long-term memory. In addition, REM is the transitional stage from the mental blankness of non-REM sleep and full wakefulness. During evolution, the increased sensitivity during the 5 or 6 periods of REM sleep was protective against danger and predators. Thus, if arousal occurs from REM sleep, the child may experience a nightmare and recall the event. In contrast to night terrors and sleep walking, Stage III sleep parasomnias are memory-less events.

In a typical night, the child will cycle between NREM and REM sleep 5 or 6 times. NREM and REM sleep occur cyclically, in varying amounts throughout the sleep period. The sleep cycle—Stages I, II, and III NREM sleep and REM sleep—will last about 50 minutes in early childhood and increase to 90 minutes in adolescence. The child will enter Stage III sleep within 10 minutes of sleep onset and stay in deep sleep for 40 to 60 minutes prior to entering REM sleep. REM sleep will only last 5 to 10 minutes early in sleep and then gradually increase in duration to 20 to 30 minutes by the fifth cycle. Stage III sleep will gradually decrease in duration during sleep and last only 10 to 15 minutes on the last cycle.

REM sleep becomes longer in duration and more intense throughout the night. As the sleep period enters the last cycles, eye movement bursts intensify along with heart rate and breathing—the most exciting dreams occur at this period of a child's sleep.

In summary, sleep is a just not the absence of wakefulness. Sleep is a dynamic state. If a disruption occurs during any of the unique sleep stage, a specific sleep disorder will be associated with this disruption.

Suggested Readings

Silber MH. Staging sleep. *Sleep Med Clin.* 2009;4(3):343-352.

Steriade M. Basic mechanisms of sleep generation. *Neurology.* 1992;42(S6):9-17.

QUESTION 4

What Changes in Breathing Are Associated With Normal Sleep?

Ritu Grewal, MD

During wakefulness, breathing is under the control of an automatic, metabolic control system located in the medulla and a voluntary or behavioral system that influences ventilation independently. This behavioral or wakefulness stimulus to breathe disappears during sleep and ventilation is entirely controlled by the medulla. The medulla has an important group of neurons called the *dorsal respiratory group* (DRG), which lies in the nucleus tractus solitarius. This is the sensory termination of the vagus and the glossopharyngeal nerve. The DRG responds to small changes in pCO_2, which diffuses through the blood brain barrier to increase ventilation. There are other groups of neurons located in the pons that influence the DRG. In addition, mechanoreceptors in the airways and lung parenchyma also influence the DRG via the vagus. When the pO_2 falls below 60 mm Hg, peripheral chemoreceptors located in the carotid bodies and aortic arch get stimulated and, via the glossopharyngeal nerve and the vagi, respectively, stimulate the DRG to increase ventilation. As ventilation increases for even small changes in pCO_2 and does not change significantly unless the pO_2 drops below 60 mm Hg in a normal, healthy person, CO_2 is the major controller of ventilation.[1]

During sleep, especially during rapid eye movement (REM) sleep, this chemo-responsiveness is reduced. In addition, there is hypotonia of both the upper airway dilator muscles and the lower respiratory muscles. Both can lead to changes in respiratory rate and rhythm, tidal volume, alveolar ventilation, and blood gases.[2]

With sleep onset, there may be a waxing and waning of respiration with emergence of central apneas. This is related to the sudden loss of wakefulness stimulus to breathe, reduced chemosensitivity at sleep onset, and transient arousal.

Minute ventilation falls during sleep—and this is primarily related to a reduction in tidal volume in adults with respiratory rate remaining relatively unchanged—except during REM sleep when it can become irregular. Studies in infants, children, and adolescents have shown that respiratory rate decreases during sleep.[3] Tidal volume and functional residual capacity decrease during sleep and these decreases are greatest during REM sleep. Both tidal volume and respiratory rate can become irregular during REM sleep with frequent emergence of central apneas.

Chidekel AS, ed. *Curbside Consultation in Pediatric Sleep Disorders: 49 Clinical Questions* (pp. 15-18)

The ensuing hypoventilation is due to a reduction of the tonic influences of wakefulness, reduced chemosensitivity, and increased upper airway resistance to airflow due to hypotonia of the upper airway dilator muscles and reduced contribution of intercostal muscles. The diaphragmatic tone is preserved relative to other respiratory muscles. Children spend more time sleeping and have more REM sleep and, accordingly, ventilation can be severely compromised, especially in neonates, for whom REM sleep can occur for up to two-thirds of total sleep time.[4]

Children have a more compliant chest wall, which causes a paradoxical inward motion during respiration with a resultant increased work of breathing, especially during sleep.[5] There is hypotonia of intercostal muscles during NREM sleep and atonia during REM sleep. The diaphragmatic tone is relatively preserved, but it is functioning close to the diaphragmatic fatigue threshold. Because of the rib cage configuration in younger children being more circular, along with reduced muscle mass, the rib cage contribution to breathing is less than that of adults. This contribution decreases drastically during sleep and, accordingly, children can decompensate more if they develop cardiopulmonary disease, especially during REM sleep.[3]

During development, the upper airway changes in both structure and function. In infants, the epiglottis may overlap the soft palate to enable them to form a better seal for suckling. This predisposes them to upper airway obstruction, especially if the nasopharynx is partly occluded. They compensate while awake by increasing the activity of the upper airway dilator muscles and increasing the respiratory rate. However, the upper airway resistance increases during sleep, especially during REM sleep, due to hypotonia of upper airway dilator muscles. Accordingly, children can develop obstructive apneas and hypopneas with nasal obstruction and enlarged tonsils and adenoids.[3]

As a result of the fall in alveolar ventilation, transcutaneous pCO_2 rises by 1 to 3 mm Hg in infants, and by 7 ± 3 mm Hg in adolescents.[3] In adults, pCO_2 increases by 2 to 8 mm Hg and pO_2 decreases by 3 to 10 mm Hg.[2] Arterial oxygen saturation (SaO_2) decreases by less than 2% during sleep in both adults and children. These changes occur despite an overall reduction of metabolism with reduced CO_2 production (VCO_2) and oxygen consumption (VO_2) in sleep.

Hypoxic and hypercapnic ventilatory responses are reduced in NREM sleep and further reduced in REM sleep. Both the oxygen response curve and the CO_2 response curve shift so that increasing amounts of oxygen desaturation (Figure 4-1) and increasing amounts of CO_2 (Figure 4-2) are needed to stimulate ventilation. The underlying mechanism is not entirely clear.[2]

Arousal responses are also reduced during sleep.[2] Arousal is an important defense mechanism to protect against hypercapnia and hypoxemia. Children have a higher arousal threshold than adults; the younger the child, the higher the threshold.[4] Hypercapnia and upper airway resistance is a stronger stimulus to arousal than hypoxemia. An increase of 6 to 15 mm Hg in pCO_2 is needed to cause an arousal, whereas SaO_2 would need to decrease to 75% before arousing a normal person. Once an arousal occurs, ventilation, including chemo-responsiveness and muscle tone, is restored to awake levels.

Central apneas are common in infants and children, particularly during REM sleep. They are considered significant if they are greater than 20 seconds in length or are associated with desaturation, bradycardia, or arousal. In contrast, obstructive apneas are uncommon. However, there are no normative data for hypopneas in children.

There is a definite decrease in VCO_2 and VO_2 with sleep onset. It increases during the early hours of the morning when REM sleep is the predominant stage. Ventilation can be severely compromised during REM sleep when the demand is at the maximum, but the output of the respiratory system is at its lowest.[2]

Laryngeal stimulation, which causes a cough reflex response, is reduced in both states of sleep and worse in REM sleep. Thus, clearance of aspirated gastric contents is reduced during sleep.

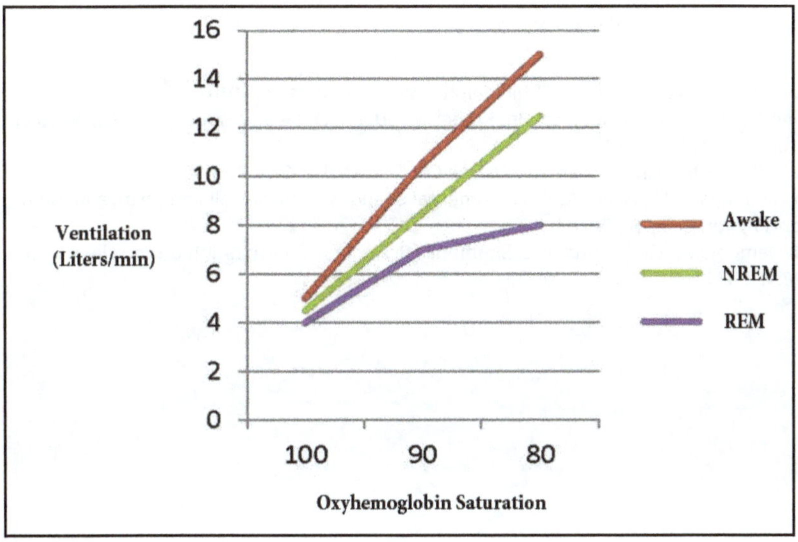

Figure 4-1. Oxygen response curve. Note reduced ventilatory response to oxyhemoglobin desaturation in sleep compared to awake state. Reduced in REM sleep compared to NREM sleep.

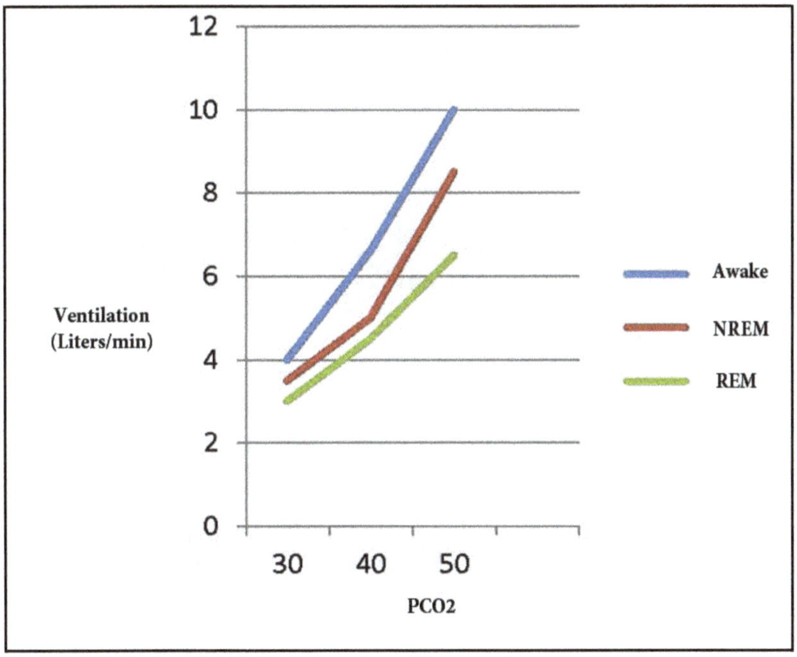

Figure 4-2. CO_2 response curve. Note reduced ventilatory response to increased pCO_2 in sleep compared to awake state. Reduced in REM sleep compared to NREM sleep.

Summary

Breathing during sleep is entirely under the influence of the automatic/metabolic controller in the medulla of the brainstem. The major cause of hypoventilation during sleep in children is reduced output from the metabolic controller with reduced respiratory rate and reduced tidal volume. Ventilation can be severely compromised during sleep, especially REM sleep in children with underlying cardiorespiratory disorders due to reduced chemo-responsiveness, hypotonia/atonia of respiratory muscles, and decreased arousal responses.

References

1. Hall JE. *Guyton & Hall Textbook of Medical Physiology*. Philadelphia: W.B. Saunders Co; 2010.
2. Krieger J. Breathing during sleep in normal subjects. In: Kryger M, ed. *Principles and Practice of Sleep Medicine*. Philadelphia: W. B. Saunders Co; 1994:212-223.
3. Marcus, CL. Sleep-disordered breathing in children. *Am J Respir Crit Care Med*. 2001;164:16-30.
4. Papastamelos C, Panitch HB, England SE, Allen JL. Developmental changes in chest wall compliance in infancy and early childhood. *J Appl Physiol*. 1995;78:179-184.
5. Carskadon MA, Harvey K, Dement WC, Guilleminault C, Simmons FB, Anders TF. Respiration during sleep in children. *West J Med*. 1978;128:477-481.

QUESTION 5

WHAT IS A CIRCADIAN RHYTHM?

Floyd Livingston, MD

The system responsible for the generation and regulation of circadian rhythms is the circadian timing system. This neural system consists of a biological clock, input pathways, and output pathways. There is substantial evidence that the paired suprachiasmatic nuclei (SCN) in the anterior hypothalamus are the site of the biological clock. The SCN are located above the optic chiasm at the base of the third ventricle. The SCN exhibit endogenous rhythmicity and have a period of oscillation close to 24 hours. The hypothalamic suprachiasmatic neurons have 3 parts that maintain the inherent rhythmicities: a way to receive input from the environment to set the clock (light, temperature); the clock (a chemical timekeeping mechanism); and genes that help the clock control the activity of the other genes. The roles of circadian clock genes in human sleep disorders have been unclear. Variations in the expression of these genes result in alterations of the circadian time period and may account for individual differences in the timing of sleep periods and arousal.

The basic molecular mechanism by which the SCN neurons generate and maintain a self-sustaining rhythm is via an auto-regulatory feedback loop in which oscillating circadian gene products regulate their own expression through a complex system of transcription, translation, and posttranslational processes. When isolated from external cues, the frequency of this oscillation (free running period) of the circadian clock is usually slightly longer than 24 hours. Light, physical activity, and melatonin keep the human circadian clock entrained in order to maintain the synchronization with the 24-hour social environment.

The SCN regulates the secretion of multiple nocturnal hormones by direct and indirect pathways, but the most important is the regulation of the secretion of melatonin—the hormone of darkness. Melatonin is produced by the pineal gland during the night in a pulsatile manner at a rate that does not vary with sleep stage. In the child, the onset of melatonin secretion occurs approximately 2 hours before bedtime at about the time of the onset of evening sleepiness. Thus, the transition phase from wakefulness and arousal to high sleep propensity coincides with the nocturnal rise in endogenous melatonin. Melatonin reaches maximum levels between 3 a.m. and 5 a.m. and decreases to low levels during the day due to suppression by light.

Chidekel AS, ed. *Curbside Consultation in Pediatric Sleep Disorders: 49 Clinical Questions* (pp. 19-20)

In contrast to melatonin, which promotes sleep, light is the giver of wakefulness and the strongest synchronizer for the circadian clock. Light will regulate the SCN through the retinohypothalamic tract that is connected with the photoreceptors in the retina. The photoreceptors provide input to the ganglion cells in the retina that contain the photo pigment melanopsin, which is most sensitive to light in the blue part of the spectrum. Blue wavelength light exposure early at night will delay circadian rhythms, pushing bedtime to a later time, while blue light in the second half of night or early morning will advance the circadian rhythm, promoting wakefulness at an earlier hour.

Almost all living organisms exhibit a circadian rhythm in their physiology and behavior. In humans, plasma melatonin, sleep/wake cycle, hormone secretion, cardiopulmonary function, cognitive performance, mood, and body core temperature show circadian rhythmicity, all of which are generated by an endogenous biological oscillator. While circadian rhythm is adjusted to 24 hours by the environmental light/dark cycle and social time cues, patients with circadian rhythm sleep disorders cannot synchronize their sleep/wake cycle to the desired time schedule and have difficulties in their social lives. Two major circadian rhythm disorders associated with insomnia are the underlying cause of sleep disruptions in such patients—delayed sleep phase syndrome and advanced sleep phase syndrome.

Circadian rhythm sleep disorders are characterized by misalignment between an individual's sleep pattern and the social norm. Parents will complain of the child's inability to fall asleep, difficulty maintaining sleep, and/or excessive daytime sleepiness. The general criteria for circadian rhythm sleep disorders, according to the *International Classification of Sleep Disorders, Second Edition,* include a persistent or recurrent pattern of sleep disturbance that is thought to be primarily due to either alteration in the circadian timing system or a misalignment between endogenous circadian rhythms and external factors that affect the timing of sleep; sleep disturbance that leads to insomnia, excessive sleepiness, or both; and sleep disturbance that is associated with impairment of function.

The 2 classic examples of circadian rhythm sleep disorders in childhood and adolescence are delayed sleep phase syndrome and advanced sleep phase syndrome. In delayed sleep phase syndrome, bedtime is pushed later into the night with corresponding later wake times that interfere with functioning, most often the ability to get to school on time. In advanced sleep phase syndrome, the circadian clock is shifted in the opposite direction with early bedtime and/or wake time that is similarly disruptive to the functioning of the child.

The sleep-wake cycle is the most important circadian rhythm in children. The regulation of the human sleep-wake cycle indicates that sleep and wake behaviors are generated by a complex interaction of endogenous circadian and sleep homeostatic processes, as well as social and environmental factors. Physiologic sleepiness and alertness not only vary with prior waking duration, but also exhibit circadian variation. The primary role of the circadian pacemaker is to promote wakefulness during the day and, thus, facilitate the consolidation of sleep during the nighttime hours.

Suggested Readings

American Academy of Sleep Medicine. Circadian rhythm sleep disorders. In: *International Classification of Sleep Disorders, Second Edition (ICSD-2).* Winchester IL: American Academy of Sleep Medicine; 2005:117-136.

Lu BS, Zee PC. Circadian rhythm sleep disorders. *Chest.* 2006;130:1915-1923.

Mongenthaler TI, Lee-Chiong T, Allesi C, et al. Practice parameters for the clinical evaluation and treatment of circadian rhythm sleep disorders. An American Academy of Sleep Medicine report. *Sleep.* 2007;30(11):1445-1459.

Panda S, Hogenesch JB, Kay SA. Circadian rhythms from flies to human. *Nature.* 2002;417:329-335.

6

QUESTION

What Are the Different Kinds of Apnea?

Floyd Livingston, MD

Central apnea occurs when there is cessation of airflow in the absence of respiratory effort. During central apnea, the polysomnogram will demonstrate the characteristic absence of naso-oral airflow, as well as thoracoabdominal movement. During an overnight sleep study, a central apnea will be scored when one of the following criteria is met:

1. The event lasts longer than 20 seconds.
2. The event lasts longer than 2 breaths and is associated either with an arousal or a dip in the oxygen saturation of 3% or more.
3. The event (in an infant) lasts longer than 2 breaths and is associated with a decrease in the heart rate to fewer than 50 beats per minute for 5 seconds or fewer than 60 beats per minute for 15 seconds.

A temporary failure or interruption in the ponto-medullary pacemaker that generates the breathing rhythm underlies central apnea. This brief absence of central nervous system output will lead to no brainstem inspiratory neural output, and the nerves innervating the inspiratory thoracic pump muscles are silent. Central apneas are quite common in normal, healthy children and adults. In fact, more than 30% of children who have been studied in clinical trials have central apneas lasting 10 to 20 seconds. This is possibly because of the overcompensation of the ventilatory response driving carbon dioxide (CO_2) levels below apnea thresholds. These heightened ventilatory responses are very active during sleep transitions from sleep to wakefulness and then back from wakefulness to sleep such that, when a child has a mild oxygen desaturation or a brief arousal, he or she tends to over-breathe to compensate and thereby drive the CO_2 below the apneic threshold, resulting in a respiratory pause while the CO_2 level rises again to the level required to stimulate breathing. Similarly, central apneas often occur while the lower waking level of CO_2 in the blood recalibrates to the higher levels associated with the sleeping apneic threshold. This is especially common in infants and young children with immature ventilatory control between wakefulness and sleep. Central apneas are seen in other conditions that affect ventilatory control, such as narcotic use or overdose, cardiac heart failure, high altitude, Arnold-Chiari malformation, acromegaly, hypothyroidism, and even obstructive sleep apnea.

Chidekel AS, ed. *Curbside Consultation in Pediatric Sleep Disorders: 49 Clinical Questions* (pp. 21-23)

Obstructive apnea is caused by an intermittent physical obstruction of the airway that impedes the flow of air through the upper airway. Obstructive apnea is characterized by an absence of airflow with continued respiratory efforts. During an overnight sleep study, an obstructive apnea will be scored if there is a 90% reduction in measured airflow despite continued respiratory effort lasting 2 breaths or longer. Because breathing against an obstructed airway is always abnormal, obstructive apneas are scored whether or not they are accompanied by an arousal, decrease in oxygen saturation, or change in heart rate.

When a child falls asleep, the upper airway narrows. If little or no air passes a site of airway obstruction—commonly the level of the tonsils—oxygen saturation may decrease, arousal may occur, and the airway will eventually reopen. The child then falls back to sleep and the normal breathing pattern resumes, and then the cycle of obstructive apnea repeats itself. The onset of an obstructive apnea occurs when forces promoting airway collapse overcome the opposing mechanisms that maintain airway patency. The airway collapse leads to increased respiratory effort in pediatric obstructive sleep apnea. Intercostal, sternal, suprasternal, and supraclavicular muscles are all recruited in severe obstructive apnea with a paradoxical inward rib cage motion during inspiration. The paradoxical motion is a desynchronization of the chest and abdominal movements instead of both the rib cage and abdomen expanding with respiration. The rib cage pulls inward due to increased negative pleural pressure generated by the recruitment of the respiratory accessory muscles and the progressive airway obstruction during an obstructive event. The abdomen still expands because of the downward motion of the diaphragm, despite increasing negative forces within the chest cavity. Enuresis is a common feature of obstructive sleep apnea caused by the increased abdominal pressure during the inspiratory phase. In contrast to central apnea, in which there is a loss of airflow secondary to airway and respiratory muscle inactivity due to lack of central nervous system output, obstructive apneas can appear quite disturbing, with the chest caving inward and the abdomen distending in the opposite direction. These forces will lead to multiple sleeping positions during the night. The child will attempt to maintain the patency of the airway with neck hyperextension, sleeping on multiple pillows, and/or chest to knee position. Sleep fragmentation will be the result of these multiple positions and post-apneic arousals. Children can experience multiple apneas per night of sleep; however, only prolonged or severe obstructive events can lead to the disruption of normal gas exchange. The sleep fragmentation and reduced REM sleep due to the multiple obstructive apneas, recorded during a polysomnogram, leads to the hallmark symptoms of daytime somnolence or hyperactivity, poor school performance, and/or behavioral consequences.

Obstructive apnea events can be caused by multiple etiologies, including tonsillar hypertrophy, adenoidal hypertrophy, enlarged tongue, anesthesia agents, and sedatives. High-risk groups that have decreased airway patency or tone (or both of these) will have increased risk of obstructive apnea, such as infants and children with obesity, Down syndrome, craniofacial syndromes, achrondoplasia, mucopolysaccharide storage diseases, and neurologic disorders.

Mixed apneas are most commonly identified by the presence of an initial central component, followed by a terminal obstructive component. Although providers might label these mixed events as obstructive, these events are pathophysiologically more similar to central apneas. A central apnea occurs because of the instability of the central controller mechanism that results in a temporary cessation of signaling to the inspiratory muscles including the upper airway muscles, upper airway caliber and tone is reduced. Airway collapse may occur and, as the child initiates breathing against a closed airway, an obstructive event follows. The mixed apneas frequently lead to brief oxygen desaturations, but are terminated by the increase of partial pressure of CO_2. In addition, more central apnea events may be seen in severe obstructive apnea as the patient attempts to overcompensate for the severe hypoxemia and breathes CO_2 below the apneic threshold. The increase in central apneas will lead to a decrease in upper airway and respiratory musculature tone, thereby causing a vicious cycle of increased obstructive events.

Summary

The diagnoses of central sleep apnea, obstructive sleep apnea, and mixed sleep apnea are made in the in-laboratory polysomnography. Central sleep apnea is characterized by a lack of drive to breathe during sleep, resulting in insufficient or absent ventilation and compromised gas exchange. In contrast, obstructive sleep has loss of airflow due to upper airway obstruction and continued respiratory excursions that will become paradoxical in severe obstruction. Mixed apnea is a combination of a central apnea followed by an obstructive event. Unrecognized and untreated apnea in childhood can lead to severe consequences, such as behavioral disorders, poor school performance, growth failure, and cardiac failure.

Suggested Readings

American Academy of Pediatrics. Clinical practice guideline: diagnosis and management of childhood obstructive sleep apnea syndrome. *Pediatrics.* 2002;109:704-712.

Berry RB, Budhiraja R, Gottlieb DJ, et al. Rules for scoring respiratory events in sleep: Update of the 2007 AASM Manual for the Scoring of Sleep and Associated Events. Deliberations of the Sleep Apnea Definitions Task Force of the American Academy of Sleep. *Clin Sleep Med.* 2012;8(5):597-619.

Eckert DJ, Jordan AS, Merchia P, Malhotra A. Central sleep apnea pathophysiology and treatment. *Chest.* 2007;131: 595-607.

QUESTION 7

What Is a Parasomnia?

Robert Heinle, MD

Sleep is often imagined as a time of rest for mind and body. This could not be further from the truth. At times during sleep, there are parts of the brain that are at least as active as they are during wakefulness. This activity determines the different sleep stages throughout the night with the most simplistic differentiation being rapid eye movement (REM) sleep, when dreaming often occurs, and non-REM (NREM) sleep. We tend to think of these stages (wakefulness, REM sleep, NREM sleep) as mutually exclusive states, but, in reality, there are times when brain activity is not distinct, particularly during transitions between sleep stages giving an overlapping picture (Figure 7-1). Parasomnias are undesirable physical events or experiences that occur during entry into sleep, within sleep, or during arousals from sleep. Parasomnias often have characteristics of both sleep and wakefulness, such as talking or movements and often occur during transitions between sleep stages.

In general, parasomnias are diagnosed by history and typically do not require extensive testing, such as a sleep study (polysomnography). The history should include such details as the time of night of occurrence, types of movements (stereotyped vs free-flowing), frequency of episodes in the night, associated fear or agitation, and whether the patient recalls the event upon awakening. Family history should be questioned for similar or other types of parasomnias. Sleep logs that document bedtime, sleep onset, parasomnias, awakenings, and time out of bed over a period of a few weeks can be helpful. Not only does this decrease recall bias of the frequency of events, but it may identify exacerbating factors, such as sleep deprivation or other stressors. The physical exam should include risks for, and evidence of, sleep-disordered breathing, such as obstructive sleep apnea, as this may also exacerbate parasomnias. The examiner should especially watch for high blood pressure, obesity, adenotonsillar hypertrophy, and micro/retrognathia. Today's technology facilitates bringing home videos of events to the physician for further review.

It is helpful to differentiate parasomnias into disorders of arousals from NREM sleep, parasomnias associated with REM sleep, and other parasomnias. Disorders of arousals from NREM sleep arise from irregularity when transitioning from slow-wave sleep to lighter stages of sleep. Because of the typical predominance of NREM sleep in the first half of the night, this is when these events often occur. These episodes are often worsened by sleep deprivation, illness,

Chidekel AS, ed. *Curbside Consultation in Pediatric Sleep Disorders: 49 Clinical Questions* (pp. 25-29)

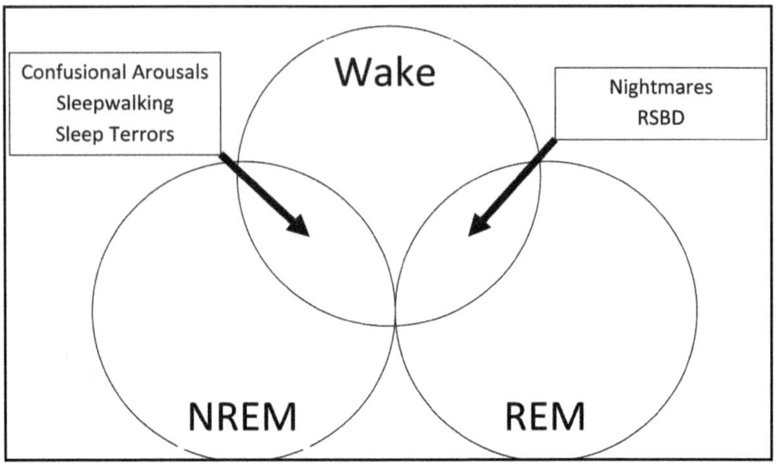

Figure 7-1. Overlapping characteristics of sleep stages leading to parasomnias. RSBD = REM sleep behavior disorder.

medications (eg, stimulants, antihistamines), obstructive sleep apnea syndrome, periodic limb movements, and gastroesophageal reflux. There may be a family history of similar events in first-degree relatives. The majority of treatment for NREM parasomnias consists of reassurance and it is the extreme exception that requires such medications as low-dose benzodiazepines. These parasomnias include confusional arousals, sleep walking, and night terrors.

Confusional arousals are classically described as moving, moaning, and crying episodes that occur a few hours after sleep onset. Although agitation is mild, there may be some verbalization of fear, such as "No" or "Go away!" Episodes may last 5 to 15 minutes and parents may become frustrated when their child is inconsolable. In fact, stimulating attempts at waking or even consoling the child may worsen agitation. Ambulation and self-injury are rare in confusional arousals. Onset is in the infant and toddler years, but prevalence may be as high as 17% in the early school years. Prevalence decreases with age down to 2% to 4% by the age of 15 years. No treatment is needed and parents should be reassured of the benign nature and self-limiting course of confusional arousals.

Sleep walking, or somnambulism, are episodes of complex, coordinated movements during sleep that may include ambulation—even going down stairs and opening doors. The child usually remains calm without signs of agitation or fear. Onset is between the ages of 5 to 10, but peaks around 11 to 12 years, with a prevalence of 17% of children this age, although only 2% to 3% will have episodes with regularity. There is often a family history of sleepwalking and the incidence of sleepwalking increases up to tenfold if a first-degree family member is affected. The main risk of sleepwalking is self-injury. There are cases of people falling down stairs, climbing through open windows, or becoming hypothermic from walking outside. The main treatment is ensuring a safe environment. If a child is a sleepwalker, windows should be closed and locked at bedtime and outside doors should have dead bolts locked. Consideration should be given to gates above stairs, or bells or alarms on the bedroom door to notify parents that the child is out of bed.

Sleep terrors are dramatic, frightening events in which a child suddenly becomes extremely agitated from sleep and does not respond to soothing measures or recall the event. These spells are usually initiated with a scream and the child seems to exhibit extreme fear or dread. There is an autonomic surge of signals from the brain, leading to a fight-or-flight response with pupillary dilatation, flushing, sweating, and tachycardia. The child is difficult to awaken. Movements may be complex, including ambulation. Onset is 2 to 10 years of age with a peak in the early school ages. Prevalence is reported at 3% to 4% in this age group and decreases to less than 1% in adults. The differential diagnosis includes nightmares (where recall is intact), nocturnal panic attacks (usually with a history of anxiety during the day), epileptic events (that occur at any time of night, repeated events throughout the night and with stereotypical movements), and cluster headaches (usually associated with unilateral periorbital pain). There is a moderate risk for self-injury and ensuring a safe environment is the mainstay of therapy.

In contrast to disorders of arousal during NREM sleep, REM-associated parasomnias typically occur in the second half of the night when REM sleep is more prevalent. REM-associated parasomnias include nightmares and REM sleep behavioral disorder; the latter occurs with the loss of muscle atonia signaling from the brainstem during REM sleep that allows the physical enactment of dreams. It is extremely rare in children, but has growing prevalence in adulthood and elderly patients. There is often combative behavior and the main safety concern is for bed partners.

Far more common in children are nightmares or extremely realistic dreams associated with fear or terror. Children often awaken from sleep agitated, but coherent, and respond quickly to reassurance and soothing measures. Recall of the dream is usually intact. There are few to no movements with nightmares and risk for self-injury is minimal. Nightmares are common in 3- to 6-year-old children, with 30% to 90% of children this age having occasional nightmares and 5% to 30% with frequent nightmares. Boys and girls are equally affected. Parents should be reassured of the benign nature of nightmares. Table 7-1 shows the differentiating characteristics of some of the common parasomnias.

Adolescents may experience a disturbing event known as recurrent isolated sleep paralysis that is a brief inability to speak or move during sleep/wake transition due to REM-sleep atonia intruding into wakefulness. Recall is intact, and hallucinations—both auditory and visual—are common. This can be an isolated event, run in families, or be associated with narcolepsy. Events may be exacerbated by fatigue, stress, alcohol, caffeine, and sleep deprivation. Onset is usually adolescence to adulthood with a 15% to 40% lifetime prevalence of at least one episode. The differential diagnosis includes atonic seizures, cataplexy, hypokalemic periodic paralysis, drug abuse/withdrawal, and hysterical/psychotic state.

Other parasomnias include a diverse group of experiences. Enuresis, or bedwetting, is a normal physiologic phenomenon in children under the age of 5 years and has decreasing prevalence with age. About 15% to 25% of 5-year-old children will continue to have enuresis that decreases to 4% to 15% of school-age children and 1% to 3% of adolescents. Enuresis is either primary, when the child never had never been consistently dry through the night, or secondary, when the child had gone at least 6 months without an episode. Primary enuresis often has a familial history. Secondary enuresis is often exacerbated by some other pathology, such as obstructive sleep apnea syndrome, urinary tract infection, constipation, diabetes, excessive evening fluid intake, ectopic ureter in females, posterior urethral valves in males, or spinal cord anomalies.

Sleep-related eating disorder has characteristics of both an eating disorder and sleepwalking. Onset is in adolescents or, less commonly, in younger children who have episodes of sleep walking and eating during the night. Particularly common are high-carbohydrate foods, although non-nutritive substances are sometimes ingested. The adolescent has no recollection of the event; however, there is usually evidence of spilled food, open cabinets, an open refrigerator, or pillows or linens in the kitchen. There is an association between sleep-related eating disorder and other parasomnias, as well as eating disorders while awake, such as anorexia nervosa or bulimia.

Sometimes noises are heard during sleep. Catathrenia is nocturnal groaning occurring in the second half of the night and may be a mild form of obstructive sleep apnea since it resolves with continuous positive airway pressure and sometimes upper airway surgery. Although not technically a parasomnia, bruxism is teeth-grinding during sleep with a prevalence of nearly half of preschool children. Mouth guards may protect teeth from damage in children with bruxism, although they do not prevent the grinding effort. There may be a false awareness of noise in exploding head syndrome, in which patients have a dramatic sensation of a painless flash of bright light and loud noise with sleep onset. Reassurance of its benign nature is the mainstay of therapy.

Table 7-1

Differentiating Characteristics of Common Parasomnias

	Confusional Arousals	*Sleep Terrors*	*Sleep-walking*	*Nightmares*	*Nocturnal Seizures*
Time of Night	First half	First half	First half	Second half	Any
Episodes per Night	1 to 2	1 to 2	1 to 2	1 to 2	Multiple
Agitation	Mild	Severe	None	Severe, improves quickly after waking	None
Movements	Mild/simple	Complex	Complex	None	Stereotyped
Out of Bed	Rare	Common	Frequent	Rare	Rare
Autonomic Surge	Minimal	Severe	None	Mild	Minimal
Recall	None	None	None	Full	Full
Risk of Injury	Low	High	High	Low	Low

Repetitive movements may be seen during sleep. Hypnic starts are isolated quick jerks of the extremities that occur near sleep onset and are seen in 70% of people of all ages. There may be an associated feeling of falling or seeing a flash of light. This is likely a release phenomenon at the level of the brainstem. Rhythmic movements are often seen in infants and toddlers during the transition from wake to sleep and typically resolve by 3 to 4 years of age. Three common types are side-to-side head rolling, head banging, and body rocking with a frequency ranging from 0.5 to 2 events per second. This is a normal occurrence and is only rarely classified as rhythmic movement disorder once self-injury occurs. The differential diagnosis includes autism and persistent developmental delay, although these etiologies often have similar recurring movements while awake. Benign neonatal sleep myoclonus consists of repetitive jerks of the extremities during the transition from wake to sleep in the first month of life. The movements cease upon awakening and resolve in weeks to months.

In general, parasomnias are benign in nature and reassurance is the only required therapy. Scheduled awakenings can sometimes help parasomnias that are frequent and recur at the same time of night. Referral to a sleep specialist should be made if there are daytime mood or behavioral disturbances, safety concerns, impaired sleep for family members, or concern for seizure disorder. Consideration for a polysomnogram should be given if parasomnias are complex or severe, or if there is evidence for obstructive sleep apnea or periodic limb movements that may be triggering parasomnias.

Suggested Readings

American Academy of Sleep Medicine. *International Classification of Sleep Disorders: Diagnostic and Coding Manual*, 2nd ed. Westchester, IL: American Academy of Sleep Medicine; 2005.

Avidan AY, Kaplish N. The parasomnias: epidemiologyclinical features, and diagnostic approach. *Clin Chest Med.* 2010;31:353-370.

Kotagal S. Parasomnias in childhood. *Sleep Med Rev.* 2009;13:e157-e168.

Mason TBA, Pack AI. Pediatric parasomnias. *SLEEP.* 2007;30(2):141-151.

National Institutes of Health. *Information About Sleep. NIH Curriculum Supplement Series [Internet]: Biological Sciences Curriculum Study.* Bethesda, MD: National Institutes of Health; 2007.

QUESTION 8

How Does Sleep Change From Infancy to Adulthood?

Mohammad Cheema, MD and Aaron S. Chidekel, MD

Sleep among newborns and young infants is polyphasic, occurring several times throughout the 24-hour day. This is distinctly different from the adult pattern of sleep, which is monophasic—occurring in one predominant sleep period during the 24-hour cycle. As an infant develops, the combination of innate developmental changes and the infant's own responsiveness to environmental cues results in sleep becoming basically monophasic, albeit with daytime naps persisting for the first several years of life. Some of these developmental factors include the maturation of the circadian timing system, general central nervous system development, and an infant's individual temperament. Important environmental cues include such factors as the infant's sleep environment, light, noise, and the general rhythms of family life.

In the first several months of their life, newborns and infants spend approximately 70% of their time asleep during the day and night (14 to 18 hours per day), although to a tired parent it does not always seem that this is possible! Later in infancy, and during the toddler years, sleep becomes even more concentrated during the overnight period, as the child continues to respond to ambient light and the sleep and activity patterns of adult caregivers and other family members. During this time period, too many distractions can certainly detract from the sleep of a toddler and the importance of a bedtime ritual and good sleep hygiene cannot be overemphasized. Total sleep time decreases and a pattern of a long overnight main sleep period with 1 or 2 daytime naps emerges (12 to 16 hours per day). Still later on in childhood, sleep time decreases further (10 to 12 hours per day) and, eventually, usually between the ages of 3 and 5 years, children give up their daytime nap altogether, which can also be a difficult time of transition for a child and family. Thereafter, a child's sleep pattern remains somewhat consistent until the innate, circadian changes and environmental challenges of adolescence can combine to favor a later bedtime and the restriction of sleep. Sleep need in adolescence is 8 to 10 hours.

The initial sleep episode in infants less than 3 months of age can be active, rapid eye movement (REM) sleep, which would be markedly abnormal in an older child or adult. There are other important differences between infant sleep patterns and more mature sleep patterns. The

Chidekel AS, ed. *Curbside Consultation in Pediatric Sleep Disorders: 49 Clinical Questions* (pp. 31-33)

proportion of NREM (Non-REM) to REM sleep is 50:50 in infants. The total sleep cycle time is short, lasting from 45 to 60 minutes. The overall percentage of REM sleep decreases with aging, from approximately 50% of total sleep time among infants to approximately 20% to 25% of total sleep time among adolescents and adults. Deep sleep (Stage N3) as a percentage of total sleep time is greatest during early childhood and declines with aging. Lastly, neonates, from birth to 2 months, are more likely to awaken from active, rather than quiet, sleep. Transitions to sleep vary during this time frame as well. Infants can fall to sleep instantly and the state-to-state transitions are short, whereas longer transitions to sleep emerge in older infants and toddlers. This can contribute to those sleep disorders related to difficulty settling both at bedtime and during normal awakenings/arousals that occur in the overnight period. Drowsiness develops during the toddler years and also results in lengthened transitions to sleep that can further contribute to sleep disorders, such as behavioral insomnia and other common sleep disorders in this age group.

In the first 6 months of life, sleep is classified into 4 sleep stages: active sleep (REM sleep-equivalent), quiet sleep (NREM sleep equivalent), indeterminant sleep, and transitional sleep. Thereafter, the more developed and differentiated pattern of NREM sleep can be recognized and scored. Active sleep first appears at 28 to 30 weeks of gestation. It is the first behavioral sleep state to appear and is the predominant sleep state in the newborn period. Active sleep is characterized by body and facial twitches and jerks, rapid eye movements, and irregular respirations. Quiet sleep is first apparent between 32 weeks (trace discontinue) and 36 weeks (trace alternant) of gestation, and it becomes the predominant sleep state by 3 months of age. *Trace discontinue* and *trace alternant* refer to the unique infantile electroencephalographic (EEG) findings associated with this stage of sleep. Other EEG characteristics of the mature sleep stages are not present at birth. Rather, sleep spindles, delta waves, and K-complexes first develop at approximately 1, 3, and 6 months, respectively. Behaviorally, quiet sleep is distinguished by its minimal or lack of body movements, regular respiration and heart rate, and the EEG patterns of high-voltage, slow-wave activity or trace alternant. Indeterminant sleep occurs if the sleep stage does not fully meet criteria for either active or quiet sleep. Transitional sleep occurs in the brief transitions between active, quiet, and indeterminant sleep.

Nocturnal sleep consolidation and sleeping through the night develops by 6 to 9 months of age. As the sleep cycle matures, the initial sleep episode is quiet (NREM) sleep, with alternating NREM and REM sleep stages. The proportion of NREM to REM sleep is roughly 75:25 among adolescents and adults, with an overall increase in NREM stage 2 sleep and a decrease in the amount of NREM stage 3 sleep occurring during this time period as well. The length of the mature sleep cycle is approximately 90 minutes in duration. The distinct EEG features that allow differentiation among the 4 stages of sleep are seen throughout the rest of an individual's lifetime. The features of NREM stage 1, NREM stage 2, NREM stage 3, and REM sleep are seen by approximately 6 months of age (Table 8-1).

As we age, the hours we sleep per day gradually decreases, averaging 14 to 18 hours in neonates (newborn to 2 months old), 12 to 16 hours in infants (2 to 12 months old), 11 to 12 hours in toddlers (1 to 3 years old), 10 to 12 hours in preschool children (3 to 5 years old), 8 to 11 hours during preadolescence (5 to 14 years old), and 7 to 9 hours during adolescence (14 to 18 years old). Generally, nocturnal sleep consolidation first develops at 6 to 9 months, and cessation of daytime napping occurs at 3 to 5 years of age. Interestingly, endogenous circadian sleep phase preference (ie, eveningness vs morningness) first develops between 6 and 12 years of age, and it is not uncommon for a sleep phase delay to emerge during adolescence—between 12 and 18 years of age.

Table 8-1

Summary of Characteristics of Mature Sleep Stages

Stage NREM 1 sleep is desynchronized (low voltage, mixed-frequency) electroencephalographic activity revealing no, or slow-rolling, eye movements and low muscle tone. Respiration and heart rate is in normal range.
Stage NREM 2 shows rhythmic electroencephalographic activity (eg, sleep spindles and K-complexes); there are still no eye movements, and reveals low muscle tone, with regular respiration and heart rate.
Stage NREM 3 reveals high voltage, slow (less than 4 Hz) frequency EEG activity, no eye movements, low muscle tone, with regular respiration and heart rate.
Stage REM is determined by desynchronized (low voltage, mixed-frequency) EEG activity with episodic rapid eye movements during phasic REM sleep and muscle atonia. The respirations are irregular along with irregular heart rate.

Summary

The first 2 years of a child's life are a time of great change in the sleep cycle and architecture of sleep. Sleep-need decreases relatively rapidly during this period of time as well, before stabilizing in early- to mid-school age. Adolescence is another time of transition in the sleep cycle as a phase shift can occur, resulting in the preference for a later bedtime and sleep onset. Sleep architecture matures in the first 6 months of life, and the components of mature REM and NREM sleep emerge as the central nervous system of an infant develops to allow for this architecture to be distinguished. With all of these rapid changes in sleep architecture and timing, it is not surprising that behavioral sleep disorders can commonly occur as a child and his or her family navigate this time of great change.

Suggested Readings

Hoban TF. Sleep and its disorders in children. *Semin Neurol.* 2004;24(3):327-340.

Jenni OG, LeBourgeois MK. Understanding sleep-wake behavior and sleep disorders in children: the value of a model. *Curr Opin Psychiatry.* 2006;19(3):282-287.

Meltzer LJ, Mindel JA. Sleep and sleep disorders in children and adolescents. *Psychiatr Clin N Am.* 2006;29:1059-1076.

Silber MH. Staging sleep. *Sleep Med Clin.* 2009;4:343-352.

SECTION II

UNIQUE ASPECTS OF SLEEP IN INFANCY

QUESTION 9

What Is Apnea of Prematurity and How Is It Treated?

Jennifer L. Maher, DO and David A. Paul, MD

Apnea of prematurity is characterized by the cessation of breathing, or airflow, and is usually accompanied by bradycardia and/or oxyhemoglobin desaturation. Its incidence increases with decreasing gestational age and it is commonly found in preterm infants less than 32 weeks of gestation and, depending on the degree of prematurity, can last through 44 weeks of corrected gestational age.

Similar to the respiratory events seen in older patients, apnea of prematurity is classified into 3 categories: central, obstructive, and mixed. Central apnea is characterized by the cessation of inspiratory effort without noted airway obstruction. Obstructive apnea occurs when there is inspiratory effort with chest wall motion; however, there is no airflow because of an obstructed upper airway. The site of upper airway obstruction is usually the pharynx, although obstruction may also occur in the larynx and, on occasion, in both sites. Mixed apnea occurs when there is a central pause with no inspiratory effort, no chest wall motion, followed by obstructed inspiratory efforts. Mixed apnea is the most common type of apnea seen in premature infants. Symptomatic apnea of prematurity of any duration occurs along a spectrum of severity and is associated with cyanosis, bradycardia, limpness, or a combination of these symptoms (Table 9-1).

Apnea of prematurity is generally thought to be a developmental disorder resulting from immaturity of the brainstem respiratory control system and should be considered a diagnosis of exclusion. When episodes increase in frequency or severity, other differential diagnoses must always be considered (Table 9-2), including bacterial infection, as sepsis often presents with worsening apnea and bradycardia events. Other diagnoses include central nervous system abnormalities, such as intraventricular hemorrhage, hypoxic ischemic encephalopathy, central nervous system malformations, seizures, hypothermia, or hyperthermia. Airway obstruction due to head positioning may also lead to apnea events in preterm infants. Anemia is frequently seen in preterm infants and can be associated with increased apnea and bradycardia events. Metabolic disorders, including hypoglycemia, hypocalcemia, and electrolyte imbalances, as well as drug effects from opiates, benzodiazepines, magnesium (generally maternal), and prostaglandins must also be considered.

Chidekel AS, ed. *Curbside Consultation in Pediatric Sleep Disorders: 49 Clinical Questions* (pp. 37-41)

Table 9-1

The Spectrum of Apnea of Prematurity Events

Mild Events

- Brief episodes
- Infrequent episodes
- Self-recovery
- Minimal or no physiological perturbation*

Moderate Events

- More prolonged events
- More frequent events
- Require stimulation to promote recovery
- Mild to moderate physiological perturbation*

Severe Events

- Prolonged events
- Frequent or clustered events
- Require intervention such as supplemental oxygen or positive pressure ventilation
- Moderate to severe physiological perturbation*

*Physiological perturbation includes oxyhemoglobin desaturation to less than 85% for greater than 5 seconds, bradycardia as defined by a decrease in heart rate by 30 beats per minute or greater, and/or a significant change in muscle tone.

Gastroesophageal reflux (GER) has been a point of contention with regard to its association with apnea of prematurity. Recent studies have shown that, although GER is found in infants with apnea, there is not necessarily a causal relationship. When looking at the timing of apnea and reflux, some data have indicated that apnea may occur first, followed by reflux.[1] The role of GER in apnea of prematurity remains an area of controversy and infants with typical GER symptoms require treatment, whereas it is unlikely that the treatment of GER will be beneficial in preterm infants with apnea alone.

Infants with apnea should be clinically evaluated. This evaluation begins with a full physical examination. The baby should receive continuous cardiorespiratory monitoring and pulse oximetry. A sepsis screen with a blood culture and complete blood count with differential (this gives an indication of sepsis as well as anemia) should be considered. Additional laboratory texts that may be done also include those relating to arterial blood gas, serum glucose, electrolytes, and calcium to evaluate for metabolic disease.

Treatment of apnea of prematurity can range from simple monitoring or basic medical therapy to airway management. Brief apneic episodes may self-resolve quickly or may resolve with tactile stimulation of the infant. The standard primary medical therapy for apnea of prematurity is caffeine (Table 9-3). Caffeine is usually given as an initial bolus to rapidly achieve a therapeutic serum level, and then as a daily maintenance dose. Caffeine therapy is typically maintained until the infant is 33 to 34 weeks corrected age. The dose should be weight-adjusted to maintain a therapeutic level. Some physicians will allow an infant to outgrow their caffeine dose. However, many

Table 9-2

Differential Diagnosis of Apnea in the Preterm Infant

Infectious Disorders

- Bacterial or viral infection
- Necrotizing enterocolitis
- Sepsis

Central Nervous System Disorders

- Intraventricular hemorrhage
- Hypoxic ischemic encephalopathy
- Seizures
- Other central nervous system malformations

Metabolic Disorders

- Anemia
- Hypoglycemia
- Hypocalcemia

Drug Effects

- Opiates
- Benzodiazepines

Miscellaneous

- Hypothermia
- Hyperthermia
- Immunizations
- Head position

Table 9-3

Caffeine Citrate for Apnea of Prematurity

Therapeutic Effects

- Increases output of respiratory center
- Increases chemoreceptor sensitivity to CO_2

Dosage

- Loading dose: 10 to 20 mg/kg IV/PO x 1
- Maintenance dose: 5 to 10 mg/kg IV/PO Q24H

clinicians believe that, if an infant requires medical treatment, it should be continued within a therapeutic range. After discontinuation, the infant should be monitored off of caffeine to observe for a recurrence of apnea/bradycardia. This monitoring period may be as long as 5 days, given the prolonged half-life of caffeine.

Caffeine treatment has been studied at length and has been found to be a safe and effective medication for the treatment of apnea. Caffeine has a wide therapeutic index. However, as with all medications, it is not without possible side effects. High levels of caffeine may result in tachycardia, cardiac dysrhythmias, feeding intolerance, diuresis, and— very infrequently—seizures. Recent randomized controlled studies were performed to evaluate concerns that there might be long-term negative side effects of caffeine treatment. These studies found that there are no associated adverse long-term neurodevelopmental or behavioral outcomes. In fact, at 2 years old, preterm infants treated with caffeine were found to have improved neurodevelopmental outcomes (reduced incidences of cerebral palsy and cognitive delay) compared to those without treatment.[2] This cohort was again evaluated at 5 years of age. Although the improved outcomes previously described with caffeine did not remain statistically significant, there was no observed harm.[3]

More clinically significant apneic events may require airway management ranging from supplemental oxygen with nasal cannula, continuous positive airway pressure (CPAP), or endotracheal intubation and mechanical ventilation. Supplemental oxygen can be used to decrease the degree of hypoxia associated with apneic episodes and, hopefully, decrease the degree of associated bradycardia. CPAP is used to stent the upper airway open and decrease the degree of airway obstruction. CPAP also helps increase the functional residual capacity of the lung, improving oxygenation and decreasing the degree of bradycardia associated with apnea. Intubation and mechanical ventilation is usually used when apnea is severe enough to lead to significant and/or recurrent bradycardia and desaturations and is unresponsive to medical therapy and less invasive airway support. When mechanical ventilation is required, the lowest possible settings should be used to decrease the degree of associated barotrauma.

Apnea of prematurity typically resolves by about 36 to 40 weeks corrected age. However, in the very premature infant (less than 28 weeks gestational age), apnea can persist through 44 weeks corrected age. Many neonatal intensive care units have a policy that infants, who are otherwise ready for discharge, should be apnea-free for 3 to 7 days before being discharged home.

In evaluating the long-term effects of apnea of prematurity, it is difficult to differentiate the causal effects of apnea alone from the independent effects of prematurity or other associated comorbidities. Because apnea events in preterm infants usually have associated bradycardia and oxygen desaturation, there is a potential causal mechanism for apnea of prematurity to lead to brain injury. Infants born very prematurely have many other significant risk factors for neurodevelopmental delays, including bronchopulmonary dysplasia, periventricular leukomalacia, or intraventricular hemorrhage. Apnea of prematurity is a common comorbidity of all of these conditions, making it difficult to determine the independent effect of apnea on long-term outcome.

The relationship between apnea of prematurity and sudden infant death syndrome (SIDS) has also been evaluated. SIDS is defined as the sudden and unexpected death of an infant less than 1 year of age, with onset of the lethal episode apparently occurring during sleep that remains unexplained after a thorough investigation, including performance of a complete autopsy and review of the circumstances of death and the clinical history. Risk factors for SIDS have been identified and include non-supine sleep position, sleeping on a soft surface, maternal smoking during pregnancy, overheating, late or no prenatal care, young maternal age, preterm birth and/or low birthweight, male gender, and African American/American or Indian/Alaskan native race. Early reports appeared to link infants with apnea to an increased risk for SIDS. More careful analysis revealed that there is unlikely to be a causal relationship between apnea of prematurity and SIDS. The peak incidence of SIDS, even in the very preterm infant, occurs at a postconceptional age when apnea of prematurity has resolved.[4]

Summary

Apnea of prematurity is a common, almost expected, complication of premature birth. It is a self-limited problem that is unique in this population and that resolves with the maturation of the respiratory control centers. Occasionally, it is the harbinger of a more significant medical problem, such as sepsis. Treatment with caffeine is usually effective for first-line therapy until the apnea resolves with development.

References

1. Corinna P. Gastroesophageal reflux and apnea of prematurity: no temporal relationship. *Pediatrics.* 2002;109(1):8-11.
2. Schmidt B. Long-term effects of caffeine therapy for apnea of prematurity. *New Engl J Med.* 2007;357(19): 1893-1902.
3. Schmidt B. Survival without disability to age 5 years after neonatal caffeine therapy for apnea of prematurity. *JAMA.* 2012;307(3):275-282.
4. Ramanathan R. Cardiorespiratory events recorded on home monitors: comparison of healthy infants with those at increased risk for SIDS. *JAMA.* 2001;285(17):2199-2207.

QUESTION 10

What Is Sudden Infant Death Syndrome?

Aaron S. Chidekel, MD

Few things are as daunting to parents or pediatric practitioners as sudden infant death syndrome (SIDS). The notion that a parent or other caregiver could place a seemingly healthy infant to sleep only to have the unthinkable happen is a source of anxiety and concern for all involved in the care of infants. Fortunately, SIDS is a rare event and there is actually quite a lot that people can do to manage the health care of mothers and infants and to improve infant sleep and the sleeping environment in order to lessen the risk that a sudden infant death will occur.

SIDS is defined as the sudden and unexpected death of an infant under the age of 1 year that remains unexplained after the examination of the death scene, the completion of a pediatric postmortem examination, and a comprehensive case review. This definition is important for its precision and specificity. An infant death prior to 28 days of life is generally considered to be a neonatal death and a death occurring after 1 year of age is no longer considered to be SIDS. The importance of a complete postmortem examination cannot be stressed enough as some causes of infant death can be subtle. Similarly, the examination of the death scene can have important safety and forensic or even legal implications. Finally, many states have special panels that convene to evaluate infant and other childhood deaths. These committees can also unmask findings with important public health and safety implications.

SIDS is an uncommon occurrence with an approximate incidence of 0.5 to 0.6 deaths per 1000 live births in the United States, an incidence that has held steady for the past several years despite great public health efforts. In addition, this global statistic does not tell the whole story, and important racial disparities remain in the incidence of SIDS just as they do for all causes of infant mortality in the United States. Table 10-1 shows SIDS rates in various groups of infants in the United States over time. Historically, SIDS rates declined significantly throughout the 1980s and 1990s, influenced by the realization that infant sleep position, specifically supine sleep, is an important modifier of SIDS risk. More recently however, SIDS rates have leveled off and clearly additional strategies are needed to reduce these rates further.

Chidekel AS, ed. *Curbside Consultation in Pediatric Sleep Disorders: 49 Clinical Questions* (pp. 43-47)

Table 10-1

Racial Disparities in Sudden Infant Death Syndrome Rates per 100,000 Live Births in the United States

	Non-Hispanic White	*Non-Hispanic Black*	*Hispanic*	*Asian and Pacific Islander*	*Overall*
1996	69.4	155.3	48.3	48.3	78.5
2006	55.6	103.8	27.0	22.8	54.5

Adapted from Taskforce on Sudden Infant Death Syndrome. SIDS and other sleep-related infant deaths: expansion of recommendations for a safe infant sleeping environment. *Pediatrics.* 2011;128:e1-e21.

Table 10-2

Selected Causes of Sudden Unexpected Infant Death

• SIDS • Accidental suffocation and strangulation in bed • Infection	• Ingestion • Metabolic disease • Cardiac channelopathy • Trauma

Although the causes of sudden unexpected infant death (SUID) are many (Table 10-2), SIDS remains the third most common cause of infant mortality, behind prematurity and congenital anomalies, and is the leading cause of infant death between the ages of 28 days and 12 months of age. Other notable medical causes of SUID include undiagnosed metabolic or cardiac conditions. Infections can strike suddenly and without warning. Unfortunately, some percentage of infant deaths are due to abuse, neglect, and infanticide. Recent attention has been given to the occurrence of accidental suffocation and strangulation in bed (ASSB). This category of SUID has been purposefully distinguished from SIDS to further highlight the risk to young infants of inappropriate sleep environments and to attempt to eliminate this preventable cause of infant death. In the past, ASSB likely overlapped with SIDS epidemiologically. As will be discussed in Question 11, a separate but proximate sleep surface in a safe and approved infant crib or bassinet is recommended for all infants to eliminate the risk of ASSB. The occurrence of these rare causes of infant deaths, which are difficult to diagnose or detect at times, highlights the importance of adhering to a strict definition of SIDS that requires a complete postmortem examination to detect a previously unsuspected condition or signs of abuse; the evaluation of the death scene to research

Table 10-3

Selected Risk Factors for Sudden Infant Death Syndrome

Infant Factors

- Premature birth
- Low birth weight
- Multiple birth
- Male sex
- Age between 1 to 4 months
- Ethnicity—particularly African American, Native American, or Eskimo
- Sibling or cousin with SIDS death

Maternal Factors

- Young mother (under 20 years of age)
- Cigarette smoking
- Other substance abuse
- Inadequate prenatal care

forensic issues and assess the occurrence of ASSB; and a comprehensive case review to evaluate the information in its entirety.

Despite many years of research, the root cause of SIDS is unknown by its very definition. Basic research has focused on central nervous system mechanisms of infant respiratory control and the genes that determine the development of the brainstem respiratory centers or other centers of autonomic control and sensory integration. Arousal responses from sleep and an individual infant's innate response to hypoxia and hypercapnia are also areas of keen interest. Examples of potential central nervous system pathways and genes include the nicotinic and serotonergic systems in the brainstem and genes, such as those related to serotonin transporter systems, brainstem development, and cardiac sodium and potassium channels. Although much of this research is either based on animal models or the retrospective analysis of infants dying of SIDS, the eventual goal is to be able to prospectively identify infants who truly are at increased risk of sudden death due to these mechanisms.

Absent a basic pathophysiologic mechanism or screening test for SIDS, the triple-risk model has served as a paradigm for the definition and management of infant sleep and risk factors for SIDS. The triple-risk model involves 3 overlapping spheres of risk: a vulnerable infant, an environmental challenge, and a physiological stress. The basic concept is that, in a vulnerable infant, an unfavorable environment and physiological stress can be combined to confront the infant with an insurmountable challenge that results in the unexpected death of the infant. By evaluating each sphere of the triple-risk model in an individual infant, a clinician can have an enormously positive impact. It is possible to define those infants who are more vulnerable or at increased risk of SIDS (Table 10-3). It is possible, but not always easy, to modify environmental risk factors to promote safety, particularly those involving safe sleep. Finally, it is also possible to ameliorate stressful situations. Modifiable risk factors for SIDS are listed in Table 10-4. For those of us in clinical practice, managing each sphere of the triple-risk model in each individual infant should be a part of our

Table 10-4

Modifiable Risk Factors for Sudden Infant Death Syndrome

Protective Factors

- Prenatal care
- Maternal health and well being
- Supine sleep in a safe crib environment
- Pacifier use
- Any breast feeding
- Immunization

Potentially Modifiable Harmful Risk Factors

- Individual impact
    - Maternal smoking during pregnancy
    - Exposure to tobacco smoke after birth
    - Parental alcohol and other substance abuse
    - Sleeping with infant on a sofa or arm chair
    - Bed-sharing
    - Overwrapping and high room temperature
    - Use of pillows, bumper pads, duvets, or loose bedding
- Public health impact:
    - Socioeconomic factors
    - Prematurity, intrauterine growth retardation, or multiple birth
    - Maternal well being

daily routines and, although it will not absolutely prevent occurrences of SIDS, it can markedly reduce the likelihood that SIDS will occur.

In clinical practice, management of the triple-risk model to reduce the risk of SIDS involves aggressive, proactive counseling and education. The most important modifiable risk factor for SIDS is sleep position, and all infants should be placed on their backs to sleep for every sleep period (supine sleep). Wakeful periods of supervised "tummy time" are also recommended. Another critically important and modifiable risk factor for SIDS is tobacco smoke exposure, both pre- and postnatally. Pregnant women should receive smoking cessation counseling and treatment; postnatally, a smoke-free zone should be maintained around infants and all children. A safe sleep surface and avoiding co-sleeping are also critical to eliminate the risk of ASSB. Other modifiable risk factors that should be discussed with families are listed in Table 10-4, and safe infant sleep and additional information about SIDS prevention are discussed in Question 11.

Summary

SIDS remains a tragedy that is not completely understood. Although SIDS remains an uncommon occurrence, practitioners should be aware of important and persistent racial disparities in SIDS rates in the United States. Adhering to the definition is critical for obvious clinical and epidemiological reasons. The lack of a basic pathophysiologic mechanism has led to the notion of the triple-risk model, which provides a useful paradigm for clinical practice and care management. A sound understanding of the epidemiology and the proactive identification and management of modifiable risk factors will help pediatric practitioners have a major impact on the health and safety of all infants for whom we provide care.

Suggested Readings

Kemp JS, Unger B, Wilkins D, et al. Unsafe sleep practices and an analysis of bedsharing among infants dying suddenly and unexpectedly: results of a four-year, population-based, death-scene investigation study of sudden infant death syndrome and related deaths. *Pediatrics.* 2000;106(3):e41.

Levene S, Bacon CJ. Sudden unexpected death and covert homicide in infancy. *Arch Dis Child.* 2004;89(5):443-447.

Neary MT, Breckenridge RA. Hypoxia at the heart of sudden infant death syndrome? *Ped Res.* 2013;74(4):375-379.

Taskforce on Sudden Infant Death Syndrome. SIDS and other sleep-related infant deaths: expansion of recommendations for a safe infant sleeping environment. *Pediatrics.* 2011;128:e1-e21.

Unger B, Kemp JS, Wilkins D, et al. Racial disparity and modifiable risk factors among infants dying suddenly and unexpectedly. *Pediatrics.* 2003;111(2):e127-e131.

Weese-Mayer DE, Ackerman MJ, Marazita ML, Berry-Kravis EM. Sudden infant death syndrome: review of implicated genetic factors. *Am J Med Genet A.* 2007;143A(8):771-778.

QUESTION 11

What Are the Latest Recommendations for Safe Infant Sleep and the Prevention of Sudden Infant Death Syndrome?

Jennifer A. Marriner, MSN, CPNP

Building on previous guidelines regarding safe infant sleep positioning, the American Academy of Pediatrics (AAP) issued further recommendations and information in 2001 in an attempt to protect babies and prevent even more infant deaths and injuries. The non-prone sleep recommendations and subsequent supine-only recommendations commencing in 1994 led to a significant reduction of approximately 50% in sudden infant death syndrome (SIDS) rates.[1] Since that time, however, there has not been any additional reduction in the number of preventable infant deaths related to sleep. It is helpful to clarify and be specific with definitions of SIDS and sudden unexpected infant death (SUID) so that they are understood by health care providers:

- SIDS—a cause assigned to infant deaths that cannot be explained after a thorough case investigation, including a scene investigation, autopsy, and review of the clinical history.[2]
- SUID—a term used to describe any sudden and unexpected death, whether explained or unexplained (including SIDS), that occurs during infancy.

It is important that we distinguish and understand definitions, as one has an unknown exact cause (SIDS), whereas the other (SUID) encompasses SIDS as well as an alarming number of preventable infant deaths. The encouraging news is that the current recommendations with regard to SIDS prevention are similar and, in some instances, the same as those that prevent or reduce the risk of all sleep-related injuries and deaths in infancy.

As was discussed in Question 10, SIDS remains a leading cause of death in infants under 1 year of age in the United States, where over 2000 infants die of SIDS each year, and about 4000 infants die suddenly with no obvious cause (SUID). A triple-risk model is theorized as a

Chidekel AS, ed. *Curbside Consultation in Pediatric Sleep Disorders: 49 Clinical Questions* (pp. 49-52)

cause of SIDS. It is thought that certain vulnerable infants are more likely to succumb during periods of critical development (usually 1 to 4 months of age) with exogenous stressors (eg, prone positioning, overheating, tobacco exposure).[3] Known risks can be easily identified and tempered with the enactment of safe sleeping practices to reduce, but not eliminate, the risk of SIDS. By contrast, the prevention of SUID, particularly with regard to sleep-related deaths and accidental suffocation and strangulation in bed (ASSB), should be enacted for all infants and can eliminate these preventable infant deaths.

There has been recognition in recent years that some deaths previously classified as SIDS are now classified as SUID and are sleep-related. Specifically classified as ASSB, these sleep-related causes of death are those linked to how or where a baby sleeps/has slept, or are related to sleep environmental hazards.[4] Accidental in nature, they include causes such as suffocation, entrapment, or strangulation. Your advice as the health care provider is an important factor in determining infant sleep-position and environment, and your advice needs to be clear, consistent, and modeled effectively. You should discuss caregiver fears regarding gastroesophageal reflux, choking, vomiting and aspiration, and sleep position that may be barriers to correct and safe practices.

Some challenges we may need to overcome when promoting safe infant sleep include the following:

- Concerns about comfort (here, it should be emphasized to parents that babies are different from children and adults)
- Conflicting advice from family members and the media
- Cultural practices and traditions
- Economic disparities

Each of these challenges can be clearly and consistently addressed in an efficient manner to ensure safe infant sleep practices. As a provider, when discussing sleep, your message should emphasize the desire to keep babies safe as something that everyone can agree is an important priority. The current AAP recommendations, which are outlined below, are divided into levels A, B, and C.[5]

- Level A recommendations are:
    - Back to sleep for all sleep time
    - A firm, safety-approved sleep surface
    - Room sharing without co-sleeping (bed-sharing)
    - No soft objects or loose bedding in the crib
    - Avoid overheating
    - Pregnant women should have regular prenatal care
    - Avoidance of tobacco exposure during pregnancy and after birth
    - Avoidance of alcohol and illicit drug use
    - Breastfeeding is recommended
    - Consider pacifier use at sleep times
    - Do not use home apnea monitors as a strategy to reduce SIDS
    - Expand the national campaign by actively involving pediatricians, family physicians, and other primary care providers to reduce the risks of SIDS with increased focus on providing a safe sleep environment

- Level B recommendations are as follows:
    - Infants should be immunized in accordance with the AAP recommendations and the Centers for Disease Control and Prevention
    - Avoid the use of commercial devices marketed to reduce the risk of SIDS
    - Supervised, awake tummy time is recommended to facilitate development and to minimize positional molding of the head
- Level C recommendations are:
    - Health care professionals, staff in newborn nurseries and neonatal intensive care units, and child care providers should model and enforce SIDS prevention recommendations beginning at birth
    - Media and manufacturers should follow safe sleep guidelines in their messaging and advertising
    - Continue research and surveillance on the risk factors, causes, and pathophysiology and mechanisms of SIDS and other sleep-related infant deaths, with the ultimate goal of eliminating all deaths entirely

These current recommendations not only stress supine-only for every sleep, but they also address the sleep environment. The "Back to Sleep" campaign has become the "Safe to Sleep" campaign/initiative to further address the environment in which babies are being placed to sleep.[6] Recommendations include that, under no circumstances, should infants sleep anywhere but in a safe space on an approved surface by themselves. Co-sleeping (or *bed-sharing*, which is now the preferred term) has not been shown to offer any protective benefits against SIDS and has been linked to SUID/ASSB. A most recent study has concluded that bed-sharing is on the rise, particularly among minorities, and the rate of bed-sharing has doubled since 1993, from 7% to 14%. This is particularly concerning as evidence is mounting that bed-sharing increases an infant's risk of death from SIDS and other sleep-related causes.[7] The perception that bed-sharing is more convenient, promotes breastfeeding, and parental closeness is just that—a perception—and it does not ensure safety. Parents who do not co-sleep with their infants are as attached and bonded to their babies and can and do breastfeed successfully. The use of armchairs and couches for feeding with a caregiver who might become tired or is already fatigued is discouraged as it has been found to be particularly hazardous. Car seats, swings, strollers, infant seats, and bouncy seats are also discouraged for infant sleeping. There is evidence that bed-sharing, as practiced in the United States and other Western cultures, is more hazardous for infants.[5]

SIDS and SUID remain public health challenges. Distinguishing between them has become increasingly more important and significant. Some causality remains unknown, but the management and recommendations with regard to modifiable risk factors are important and impactful. Current recommendations, if they are clear, promoted, and practiced, are meaningful and save lives.

References

1. National Infant Sleep Position. *http://slone-web2.bu.edu/chimenisp/main_nisp.asp*. Accessed October 10, 2013.
2. Willinger M, James LS, Catz C. Defining the sudden infant death syndrome (SIDS): deliberations of an expert panel convened by the National Institute of Health and Human Development. *Pediatr Pathol.* 1991;11(5):677-684.

3. Filiano JJ, Kinney HC. A perspective on neuropathologic findings in victims of the sudden infant death syndrome: the triple-risk model. *Biol Neonate*. 1994;65(3-4):194-197.
4. Schnitzer PG, Covington TM, Dyskstra HK. Sudden unexpected infant deaths: sleep environment and circumstances. *Am J Public Health*. 2012;102(6):1204-1212.
5. Task Force on Sudden Infant Death Syndrome, Moon RY. SIDS and other sleep-related infant deaths: expansion of recommendations for a safe sleeping environment. *Pediatrics*. 2011;128(5):1030-1039.
6. Eunice Kennedy Shriver National Institute for Child Health and Human Development, NIH, DHHS. *Safe Sleep for Your Baby: Reduce the Risk of Sudden Infant Death Syndrome (SIDS) and Other Sleep-Related Causes of Infant Death (12-7040)*. Washington, DC: U.S. Government Printing Office; 2012.
7. Colson ER, Willinger M, Rybin D, et al. Trends and factors associated with infant bed sharing, 1993-2010: the National Infant Sleep Position Study. *JAMA Pediatr*. 2013;167(11):1032-1037.

QUESTION 12

What Is an Apparent Life-Threatening Event?

Amy Renwick, MD

The occurrence of apparent life-threatening events (ALTEs) is a fairly common infant problem, accounting for about 1% of pediatric emergency room visits and 2% of inpatient admissions. ALTE was defined in an National Institutes of Health consensus statement as "an episode that is frightening to the observer and that is characterized by some combination of apnea (central or occasionally obstructive), color change (usually cyanotic or pallid, but occasionally erythematous or plethoric), marked change in muscle tone (usually marked limpness), choking, or gagging."[1] ALTE is more common among premature infants and young infants, and affects males and females equally. Overall mortality rates are low: 0% to 0.6% in most published series.

Note that the ALTE literature must be interpreted with caution—subjectivity is inherent in the definition and the criteria are quite broad, so the term may be applied variably from one practitioner or institution to another. Some studies excluded patients for whom a cause was obvious at the time of presentation or determined later, and others did not.

Because ALTE is a descriptive term rather than a diagnostic one, the clinician is faced with the challenge of how to proceed in the evaluation of an infant with an ALTE. In many cases, no clear etiology is found, and in many others a possible cause is suggested, although the true association with the event may not be certain. For instance, because gastroesophageal reflux (GER) is very common in all infants, it is also common among infants with ALTE, so the finding of GER does not demonstrate that GER was the cause of an ALTE.

The basic workup for any infant presenting with an ALTE is a detailed history as outlined in Table 12-1, and a careful physical examination. Whenever possible, one should obtain history from witnesses to the event, any first-responder and/or emergency room reports, and the infant's usual caregivers. Try to determine if the event happened while the infant was awake or asleep. Ask about the appearance and activity of the infant during the event, the preceding circumstances, and the duration of the event itself and any subsequent differences from baseline. If there was intervention, assess exactly what was done, whether it seemed to have been truly necessary, and the child's response. Take a full medical history, asking particularly about any previous similar events, and family history, especially regarding any infant deaths.

Chidekel AS, ed. *Curbside Consultation in Pediatric Sleep Disorders: 49 Clinical Questions* (pp. 53-57)

Table 12-1

Important Elements of the History

- A detailed description of the infant during the event, including:
  - Was there cyanosis (differentiate central cyanosis from peripheral or perioral)?
  - Choking?
  - Any apparent respiratory effort?
  - Rhythmic movement, twitching, or eye deviation?
- The circumstances leading up to the event (time and content of last feeding, position of infant, who was caring for the infant at the time and during the several hours before the event, etc)
- Any fever? Other signs or symptoms of illness?
- Whether there was a true need for resuscitation (keep in mind that it may have been started at home without an assessment)
- Whether the infant has returned to baseline and, if so, how long that took
- Whether there have been previous events and, if so, their frequency and whether there has been any change in frequency, severity, or character
- General growth, development, birth, and past medical history
  - Family history, with attention to the following:
    - Miscarriages
    - Stillbirths and infant or child deaths
    - Seizures and cardiac disease
- Results of newborn screening and any other previous studies
- Whether the child was given any of the following:
  - Medications
  - Supplements
  - Inappropriate foods

A complete physical examination should be performed, including vital signs, oxygen saturation, assessment of growth parameters, a thorough neurologic exam, and close inspection for signs of trauma.

Child abuse deserves special mention, as it is not uncommon as a cause of ALTE, and the potential for subsequent morbidity or mortality is high. In one study, historical factors that were associated with abuse were vomiting, irritability, or a 911 call. Many of the earlier studies of infant ALTE did not take child abuse, factitious illness, or Munchausen syndrome by proxy into consideration, particularly in cases of recurrent ALTE. Any inconsistencies in the history should also increase your suspicion for abuse.

Testing should be guided by information from the history, physical exam, and clinical course as the differential diagnosis of ALTE is quite broad (Table 12-2). Although most babies with ALTE will have a benign course, a minority will have truly life-threatening conditions—and

Table 12-2

Differential Diagnosis

Gastrointestinal

- Gastroesophageal reflux
- Dysphagia
- Laryngeal chemoreflex apnea

Respiratory

- Respiratory syncytial virus or other viral infection
- Pertussis
- Laryngomalacia

Neurologic

- Seizure
- Intracranial hemorrhage
- Apnea of Infancy

Cardiac

- Arrhythmia
- Congenital heart disease

Metabolic

- Hypoglycemia
- Electrolyte disturbance
- Inborn error of metabolism

Sepsis

Child Abuse

- Shaken baby syndrome
- Intentional suffocation
- Munchausen syndrome by proxy

Miscellaneous

- Periodic breathing
- Acrocyanosis
- Breath-holding spell
- Accidental suffocation strangulation in bed
- Idiopathic

Adapted from DeWolfe CC, Chidekel AS, Apparent life-threatening event, infant apnea and pediatric obstructive sleep apnea. In: Zaoutis LB, Chiang VW. *Comprehensive Pediatric Hospital Medicine.* Philadelphia: Mosby Elsevier; 2007:453-462.

Table 12-3

Workup

Basic

- History
- Physical exam
- Directed studies as suggested by information from the history and physical
- Period of clinical observation with pulse oximetry

Second-Line

- CBC with differential
- Electrolytes
- Blood glucose
- Tests for pertussis and respiratory syncytial virus
- Urine culture, urinalysis
- Urine toxicology screen
- Head CT scan or brain MRI
- Chest x-ray
- Skeletal survey
- Electrocardiogram, with consideration for longer rhythm monitoring
- Electroencephalogram
- Feeding evaluation
- Dilated eye exam
- Pneumogram/polysomnogram

CBC = Complete blood count; CT = Computerized tomography; MRI = Magnetic resonance imaging.

the 2 groups can be very difficult to distinguish. There are no standard panels of tests that have been shown to be reliable in determining the cause of an ALTE, the need for admission, or the likelihood of a poor outcome. A stepwise approach to ALTE is briefly outlined in Table 12-3.

In cases in which the history and physical exam are not contributory, investigations with a relatively high diagnostic yield include urinalysis, urine culture, neuroimaging (brain magnetic resonance imaging or head computerized tomography scan), pneumogram, or polysomnogram, chest x-ray, and white blood cell count.[1] Other studies that are fairly easy to obtain and may reveal important information are an electrocardiogram, Bordetella pertussis and RSV testing, blood glucose and electrolytes, blood culture, and urine toxicology screen. Although seizures are a significant cause of ALTE, an electroencephalography at the time of presentation often is not diagnostic.

Pneumograms or polysomnography may be useful for gathering complete data on heart rate, respiratory patterns, and oxygen saturation over many hours. It may identify exaggerated periodic breathing. If an event occurs during the study, it can demonstrate any heart rate abnormalities and their temporal relationship to respiratory changes, and distinguish central from obstructive and mixed apnea.

I seldom pursue testing specifically to identify GE reflux, but if the history is suggestive then I usually institute reflux precautions and would consider medication.

No additional workup may be needed for a single episode in an afebrile, previously well, term infant who did not require resuscitation, has returned to baseline, appears well, and has normal vital signs and exam.

Management, of course, depends on the underlying cause, if it is determined. A period of observation is prudent, particularly if intervention was required. Although not all infants with uncomplicated ALTE require admission, I generally keep uncomplicated patients until about 24 hours after the event. Monitoring during this period should include at least heart rate, respiratory rate, and oxygen saturation and be started promptly so that any further events are captured.

I generally suggest infant cardiopulmonary resuscitation training for parents and other caregivers so they feel more prepared for any future events. The family should be watched for any changes in feeding, breathing, or alertness and one should follow up closely with the primary care provider. Families can be reassured that ALTE and SIDS are separate entities. As discussed in Question 11, safe sleep practices should be reviewed.

Many families have questions about the need for home monitoring after an ALTE. The use of home apnea monitors will be discussed in Question 13. Short-term home cardiorespiratory monitor use may be appropriate in cases of known or suspected central apnea, or for unexplained, but severe events. If there is concern for significant obstructive apnea with oxygen desaturation, pulse oximetry can be used instead. Both are likely to have frequent false alarms, particularly in more mobile infants. Home monitoring has not been demonstrated to improve outcomes in general populations of infants with ALTE.

References

1. Brand DA, Altman RL, Purtill K, et al. Yield of diagnostic testing in infants who have had an apparent life-threatening event. *Pediatrics* 2005;115:885-893.

Suggested Readings

Kahn A. Recommended clinical evaluation of infants with an apparent life-threatening event: consensus document of the European Society for the Study and Prevention of Infant Death, 2003. *Eur J Pediatr.* 2004;163:108-115.

McGovern MC, Smith MB. Causes of apparent life threatening events in infants. A systematic review. *Ach Dis Child.* 2004;163:108-115.

National Institutes of Health. *Infantile Apnea and Home Monitoring.* Bethesda, MD: National Institutes of Health; 1986.

QUESTION 13

What, if Anything, Are Apnea Monitors Used For?

Vanessa Shanks, MD and David A. Paul, MD

Home monitoring remains a controversial clinical topic. Despite extensive research, the pathophysiology of sudden infant death syndrome (SIDS) remains unclear. Premature infants, siblings of SIDS victims, and term infants who have experienced an apparent life-threatening event (ALTE) are thought to be at greatest risk of SIDS. Unfortunately, no study has been able to demonstrate that intervening with home monitoring saves the lives of these infants. In this chapter, we will examine each of these patient populations to help delineate the appropriateness of home monitoring in each situation.

Apnea of prematurity, a developmental process that results from immature respiratory centers in the brain, is not believed to be an independent risk factor for SIDS. Although it can cause great frustration for both medical providers and parents when persistent apnea prevents an infant's discharge from the hospital, it is a temporary condition that often resolves by 44 weeks' postconceptional age. The margin of safety for hospital discharge has not been extensively studied. One study showed institutional variability in discharge policies and suggested that, if an infant has not experienced apnea within 8 days of a previous episode, the infant is unlikely to do so in the future.[1]

Some hospital policies substitute home monitoring in place of an apnea-free period to facilitate earlier home discharge. Unfortunately, in 2001, the Collaborative Home Infant Monitoring Evaluation, or CHIME, study showed that all infants had episodic apnea and bradycardia, including healthy term infants; however, this study was unable to demonstrate any correlation between these episodes and infant death.[2] The American Academy of Pediatrics (AAP) subsequently released a policy statement that concluded that episodic apnea was not an immediate precursor to SIDS and that home cardiorespiratory monitoring was not an effective tool to prevent SIDS.[3] Home cardiorespiratory monitoring may be beneficial in those infants discharged with home oxygen or on ventilator support since desaturation events in these infants may be attributable to mechanical malfunction that can be intervened upon. Pulse oximetry is often used in these cases as well, and the AAP policy statement does not specify which monitoring system is most appropriate.

Chidekel AS, ed. *Curbside Consultation in Pediatric Sleep Disorders: 49 Clinical Questions* (pp. 59-61)

The risk of recurrence in subsequent siblings of SIDS victims is also controversial. As the epidemiology of SIDS has become better understood, the clinical practice of monitoring siblings of SIDS victims has changed. Previous studies that reported an increased risk or recurrence of SIDS had not taken into account the importance of infant sleeping position and sleeping environment, the presence of smoking in the household, and the importance of death scene investigation. These studies also had not considered the role of infanticide or induced illness in the medical setting (Munchausen syndrome by proxy). These significant forensic and environmental factors make it difficult to determine the true recurrence risk posed to siblings of SIDS victims. The AAP policy statement, which addresses the use of home monitors in the premature infant, states that the true risk of recurrence of SIDS in siblings is unclear, but it is most likely exceedingly low.[3] The efficacy of home monitoring in this population also remains unproven, despite several studies attempting to do so; therefore, the AAP does not recommend the use of home cardiorespiratory monitors as a means of preventing SIDS in siblings of SIDS victims. Based on more recent studies, the AAP made the following recommendations, in addition to supine sleeping, which appear to also decrease the risk of SIDS: the use of a firm sleep surface; breastfeeding; room-sharing without bed-sharing; consideration of a pacifier; and the avoidance of overheating and exposure to tobacco, smoke, alcohol, and illicit drugs should be encouraged for all infants.[4]

Term infants who experience an ALTE are a poorly defined group since the diagnosis is based on subjective symptoms as reported by the caregiver. Most infants who experience an ALTE recover from the initial event and survive. However, there is no evidence as to the risk of recurrent events or subsequent death. Despite undergoing diagnostic testing in the hospital setting, up to 50% of infants who experience an ALTE are discharged home without a known cause for their symptoms. Home cardiorespiratory monitoring has not been shown to be effective at preventing SIDS in this population; however, monitors with memory capability have been shown to be helpful in establishing a diagnosis in infants with recurrent ALTE and an unremarkable initial evaluation, including seizures, arrhythmias, suffocation, and induced illness in the medical setting or Munchausen syndrome by proxy.[5] For this reason, the AAP recommends that consideration of home cardiorespiratory monitoring be prescribed on an individualized basis with the intent of obtaining a diagnosis, but not preventing SIDS.[3] If a clinician decides to employ home cardiorespiratory monitoring, it should have an event recorder and the settings should be physiologically appropriate (Table 13-1) and close follow-up including family support should be maintained throughout the period of monitoring.

Table 13-1

Age-Appropriate Cardiorespiratory Monitor Settings

Condition	*Setting Threshold*
Apnea	
• Premature infants	15 seconds
• Full-term infants	20 seconds
Bradycardia	
• Premature infants	
○ Postconceptional age < 40 weeks	100 beats per minute
○ Postconceptional age 40 to 44 weeks	80 beats per minute
○ Postconceptional age > 40 weeks	Use full-term values for corrected age
• Full-term infants	
○ < 1 month	80 beats per minute
○ 1 to 3 months	70 beats per minute
○ 3 to 12 months	60 beats per minute
○ > 12 months	50 beats per minute
Tachycardia	
• All infants	220 beats per minute

Adapted from DeWolfe CC, Chidekel AS. Apparent life-threatening event, infant apnea and pediatric obstructive sleep apnea. In: Zaoutis LB, Chiang VW, eds. *Comprehensive Pediatric Hospital Medicine.* Philadelphia: Mosby Elsevier; 2007:453-462.

References

1. Darnall R, Kattwinkel J, Nattie C, Robinson M. Margin of safety for discharge after apnea in preterm infants. *Pediatrics.* 1997;100:795.
2. Ramanathan R, Corwin MJ, Hunt CE, et al. Cardiorespiratory events recorded on home monitors: comparison of healthy infants with those at increased risk for SIDS. *JAMA.* 2001;285(17):2199-2207.
3. Committee on Fetus and Newborn. American Academy of Pediatrics. Apnea, sudden infant death syndrome, and home monitoring. *Pediatrics.* 2003;111(4 Pt 1):914-917.
4. Task Force on Sudden Infant Death Syndrome, Moon RY. SIDS and other sleep-related infant deaths: expansion of recommendations for a safe infant sleeping environment. *Pediatrics.* 2011;128(5):1030-1039.
5. Silvestri JM. Indications for home apnea monitoring (or not). *Clin Perinatol.* 2009;36(1):87-99.

SECTION III

NONRESPIRATORY SLEEP DISORDERS OF INFANCY AND CHILDHOOD

QUESTION 14

My Infant Just Won't Sleep. What Are Some Common Sleep Disorders Unique to Infants?

Persephone Jones, MD, MPH and Rhonda Walter, MD

Sleep problems are a common complaint of parents of infants in pediatric practice. Most sleep problems encountered in infants are related to difficulty falling asleep and staying asleep throughout the night. It is estimated that bedtime problems and frequent night wakings occur in 10% to 30% of children over 6 months of age.[1,2] Infant sleep problems can have a significant impact not only on infants, but on their parents and family members.

Identification of sleep disorders in infants can be challenging as normal sleep patterns rapidly evolve. In newborns, the focus is primarily on feeding and weight gain. Feeding occurs at least once every 3 to 4 hours, or even more often in breastfed babies. Therefore, although newborns spend approximately 16 hours per day sleeping, their sleep is frequently disrupted to feed, and this disruption is normal and expected. In addition, newborn sleep is often evenly divided between day and night, or there can even be some confusion of day and night cycles. Once weight gain has been established, increased consolidation of nighttime sleep should occur. Between 1 and 3 months of age, the amount of time that babies are able to sleep without feeding increases and they begin to settle into a sleep routine. By 4 to 7 months of age, babies may be sleeping up to 7 or 8 hours at night, plus taking 2 to 3 naps, for a total of approximately 14 hours. Many babies are sleeping through the night by 6 months of age or sooner; however, 25% to 50% of children older than 6 months of age continue to awaken during the night.[3] Once a child begins to sleep through the night, though, there can be regressions in sleep, which may worsen during times of rapid developmental change and acquisition of milestones (eg, awakening to practice a new skill). There can also be worsening in the ability to sleep through the night between 8 and 12 months of age due to separation anxiety, a normal developmental milestone. Parental (or caregiver) response to these normal developmental changes in sleep can result in a number of sleep problems that are unique to infants and young children. These are listed in Table 14-1 and can be addressed with a combination of supportive parenting skills and the behavioral techniques introduced next.

Chidekel AS, ed. *Curbside Consultation in Pediatric Sleep Disorders: 49 Clinical Questions* (pp. 65-68)

Table 14-1

Behavioral Sleep Problems Unique to Infants

- Colic
- Delayed settling
- Trained night feeding
- Trained night awakening
- Developmental night awakening

Differences in infant sleep have both a genetic and environmental component.[4] There is significant variation in sleep needs in children of the same age. There are also temperamental variations that can have a significant influence on sleep. Infants present with differences around levels of fussiness and also in their ability to self-soothe. Environmental influences on sleep include the physical environment for sleep and parent characteristics. Some parents have a greater tendency to perpetuate sleep associations that can have a negative effect on sleep. Medical and physiologic conditions may also have a negative effect on sleep. Common infant conditions such as colic, gastroesophageal reflux, otitis media, atopic dermatitis, and teething can negatively impact sleep. Treatment of these medical problems can help sleep. In addition, children who have neurological disorders or neurodevelopmental disabilities are significantly more likely to present with sleep problems. Sleep challenges in children with medical issues may also be exacerbated by parental difficulties in setting limits due to perceived vulnerability of the child.

Sleep disorders are defined as either medical (associated with abnormal polysomnography) or behavioral. The majority of sleep disorders in infants are behavioral. In 2005, the *International Classification of Sleep Disorders* introduced a diagnostic category of behavioral insomnia of childhood. This category includes both sleep onset association and limit-setting subtypes.[5] In order to diagnose a sleep disorder, the symptoms must have been occurring for a specific amount of time and result in impaired functioning in the child or other family members. There are many important factors to consider when evaluating for the presence of a sleep disorder. A child's developmental level and reasonable expectations for sleep at that developmental level must be considered. There is also some significant variability between families regarding what is accepted as normal sleep; a sleep pattern that is problematic for one family may be acceptable for another. It is important to ensure that expectations for sleep are appropriate for a child's age and that they are not being expected to sleep at a time when they are simply not tired or for longer than they are capable of sleeping. However, children should be provided the opportunity to get all the sleep that they require. It is a common misconception that preventing babies from napping or missing naps will help them to sleep by "tiring them out." In fact, the opposite is true; when a baby is overtired, he or she is less likely to sleep well at night.

The sleep association subtype of behavioral insomnia is extremely common in infants and is very treatable. In this disorder, an infant has specific sleep associations, typically requiring parental intervention, in order to fall asleep. Examples of sleep associations include being held, rocked, or fed. During sleep, there are normal brief arousals occurring at the end of each sleep cycle. If an infant requires specific sleep associations to fall asleep, he or she will not be able to fall back to sleep independently (self-soothe) when these arousals occur. Instead, he or she will awaken and cry out to the caregiver in order to signal them to provide the association necessary to fall asleep again. Development of sleep associations can be avoided by teaching infants to fall

Table 14-2

Management of Sleep Onset Association Behavioral Insomnia

Unmodified Extinction	*Graduated Extinction*	*Scheduled Awakenings*
• "Cold turkey" approach • Put child to bed at designated bedtime and ignore all crying/protest until a specified time the next morning • Very effective • Very difficult for parents to tolerate • May see improvement within a few days	• "Sleep training" or "Ferber method" • Put child to bed "drowsy but awake" • Use of a fixed or progressively longer interval schedule tailored to patient's age, temperament, parental tolerance • Minimize interactions during check-ins • Initially use check-ins for bedtime only; later, generalization to nighttime awakenings • Improvement in approximately 1 week if consistently used	• Awakening and consoling child 15 to 30 minutes prior to expected awakening • Parent-induced awakening followed by parents' usual response such as nursing or rocking to sleep • Scheduled awakenings faded out by increasing amount of time between awakenings • Improvement may take weeks

asleep independently by putting them to bed while they are drowsy, but still awake. Parents can also address sleep associations by allowing their child a few minutes to self-soothe when they cry out rather than rushing to their baby to intervene. Often, after crying for a few minutes, infants can soothe themselves and fall asleep without any further intervention. It is important to ensure that all of a child's physiologic needs have been met—in other words, that they do not have a dirty diaper, are not ill, and are not uncomfortable in any other way. If an infant requires tending to at night, for example, so that he or she can be fed or so that a diaper can be changed, this should be performed in a way that is as brief and non-stimulating as possible in order to convey the message that nighttime is for sleep. Keeping the lights low and other forms of stimulation to a minimum are simple starting points.

Behavioral interventions for management of sleep onset associations can be very effective and include unmodified extinction, graduated extinction and scheduled awakenings[6] (Table 14-2). Unmodified extinction consists of allowing children to "cry it out." With this method, parents put a child to bed at a designated bedtime and ignore the child's crying and protest until a set time in the morning. While this is very effective, it is very difficult for most parents. In graduated extinction, parents ignore bedtime crying and tantrums for specific and increasing periods of time. This method is frequently referred to as the "sleep training" or the "Ferber method." Scheduled awakenings is a third method that is used to help children to sleep through the night. This involves waking children 15 to 30 minutes before the typical wake time and providing the usual sleep association. Over time, this can be helpful in reducing nighttime awakenings. It may be helpful for families who are not comfortable allowing their infant to cry at night.

Establishment of a routine early on is also very helpful in fostering sleep. This routine does not need to be elaborate, but it should be consistent. For example, a routine can include feeding, a bath, a bedtime story, or a lullaby. The bedtime routine signals to a child that the time for sleep is approaching. The more a routine has been established, the easier it is to get sleep back on track after disruptions to the routine, such as during illness or family stressors. The sleep environment is also very important. In order to promote self-soothing and decreased dependence on sleep associations, children should fall asleep in a safe place, such as a crib rather than in their parents' arms or a swing, which can contribute to sleep association problems and decreased quality of sleep. It is also important that the sleep environment not be too warm or too cold.

Although infant sleep problems are often very stressful for families, they are most often behavioral and can be significantly improved with attention to scheduling, routine, consistency, and elimination of sleep associations. These modifications can have significant results even in "difficult" sleepers. Providing support and guidance to families during this trying time can often have very satisfying results.

References

1. Byars KC, Yolton K, Rausch J, Lanphear B, Beebe DW. Prevalence, patterns and persistence of sleep problems in the first 3 years of life. *Pediatrics.* 2012;129(2):e276-e284.
2. Mindell, JA, Kuhn BR, Lewin DS, et al. Behavioral treatment of bedtime problems and night wakings in infants and young children. *Sleep.* 2006;29:1263-1276.
3. Mindell JA, Owens JA. *Clinical Guide to Pediatric Sleep: Diagnosis and Management of Sleep Problems.* Philadelphia: Lippincott Williams & Wilkens; 2003.
4. Fisher A, van Jaarsveld CHM, Llewellyn, CH, Wardle, J. Genetic and environmental influences on infant sleep. *Pediatrics.* 2012;129(6)1091-1096.
5. American Academy of Sleep Medicine. *International Classification of Sleep Disorders: Diagnostic and Coding Manual,* 2nd ed. Westchester, IL: American Academy of Sleep Medicine; 2005.
6. Morgenthaler TI, Owens J, Alessi C, et al. Practice parameters for behavioral treatment of bedtime problems and night wakings in infants and young children. *Sleep.* 2006;29(10):1277-1281.

Suggested Readings

Ferber R. *Solve Your Child's Sleep Problems.* New York: Simon and Schuster; 2006.

Weissbluth M. *Healthy Sleep Habits, Happy Child.* New York: Ballantine Books; 2005.

QUESTION 15

What Are Nightmares?

Robert Heinle, MD

Only about 1 in 10 people have never had a nightmare. Vivid dreams of being chased, falling, or surrounded by snakes or other monsters may terrorize and disrupt our sleep, but what are these events that leave us awake, sweating, and panicked in the early morning hours? To understand nightmares, one needs to understand some basic physiology of sleep. As detailed in Question 7, parasomnias are undesirable physical events or experiences that occur during entry into sleep, within sleep, or during arousals from sleep. Parasomnias often have characteristics of both sleep and wakefulness, such as talking or movements and often occur during transitions between sleep stages. Nightmares are a specific example of a parasomnia that occurs when a child has an extremely realistic dream associated with fear or terror. Because dreams occur during rapid eye movement (REM) sleep that is predominantly in the latter part of the night, these episodes typically happen in the second half of the night.

Common in childhood, nightmares are episodes of vivid, disturbing dream activity that often become progressively more intense until they trigger a full awakening from REM sleep in the early morning hours of the second half of the night. Children often awaken from sleep agitated but coherent, and respond quickly to reassurance and soothing measures. Episodes are usually brief in duration. Muscle atonia associated with REM sleep remains in place, resulting in little to no movement during nightmares and, therefore, the risk for self injury is minimal. Mild tachycardia may be present but, as opposed to night terrors, other signs of autonomic surge (eg, pupillary dilatation, flushing) are minimal or absent. Recall of the dream is usually intact and this may delay the ability to return to sleep.

Nightmares are most common in 3- to 6-year-old children, with 30% to 90% of children this age having occasional nightmares and 5% to 30% having frequent nightmares. This is also the time of childhood when general bedtime fears are most common. Boys and girls are equally affected and this differs from adults as women are more likely to have nightmares than men. As opposed to other parasomnias, nightmares persist into adulthood, with nearly 85% of adults reporting at least one nightmare in the previous year, although weekly nightmares are only present in 2% to 6% of adults. Studies have suggested a strong genetic role in determining the frequency and severity of

Chidekel AS, ed. *Curbside Consultation in Pediatric Sleep Disorders: 49 Clinical Questions* (pp. 69-71)

Table 15-1

Management of Nightmare Disorder

- Simple management
  - Reassurance/rescripting
  - Bedtime ritual and security object to prepare for good dreams
  - Brief intervention in child's room
  - Avoid secondary gain
- Complex management
  - Counseling
  - Relaxation techniques
  - Medical therapy

nightmares in twins and families. Children who have been sexually abused or diagnosed with posttraumatic stress disorder may have nightmares that relive the events or dreams about non-specific threatening situations. Nightmare disorder associated with these unfortunate occurrences will require more intensive and multidisciplinary treatment. Watching violence on television may also contribute to anxiety-provoking dream content, especially if this occurs just prior to bedtime. Anxiety disorders and posttraumatic stress disorder in adolescents have both been associated with increased frequency of nightmares.

The differential diagnosis for nightmares includes night terrors and REM-sleep behavior disorder (RSBD). During episodes of night terrors, children are typically inconsolable, with complex movements including ambulation, and afterwards have no recollection of the event. RSBD is extremely rare in young children, although onset may occur in adolescence, and episodes include prominent complex movements as the patient physically acts out the dream, often including combative behaviors. Patients with RSBD will recall the dream fully and describe the actions they were performing.

Diagnosis is usually made by history and does not typically require such testing as polysomnogram. A basic treatment approach to nightmares is outlined in Table 15-1. Parents should be reassured of the benign nature of nightmares. Reassurance, a familiar and comforting bedtime ritual, and a transitional object are often all that is required after simple nightmares. Rescripting, in which parents and children alter the nightmare into a dream with a more pleasant ending, may also be helpful. Desensitization by discussing or drawing scenes from nightmares during the day has been shown to decrease the fear associated with nightmares. Avoiding exacerbating factors, such as violent experiences (eg, television, video gaming), for 2 hours prior to sleep is sometimes recommended.

Summary

Nightmares are common parasomnias seen in both children and adults where intense dreams associated with fear/dread increase to a full awakening with accurate recall of events and good response to soothing, consoling technique, and little risk of self-injury. Limiting intense experiences prior to bed, rescripting, and desensitization are all techniques to reduce fear and severity associated with nightmares. In the end, parental reassurance of the benign nature of nightmares forms the basis of therapy.

Suggested Readings

American Academy of Sleep Medicine. *International Classification of Sleep Disorders: Diagnostic and Coding Manual,* 2nd ed. Westchester, IL: American Academy of Sleep Medicine; 2005.

Mason TBA, Pack AI. Pediatric parasomnias. *SLEEP.* 2007:30(2);141-151.

Avidan AY, Kaplish N. The parasomnias: epidemiologyclinical features, and diagnostic approach. *Clin Chest Med.* 2010;31:353-370.

Kotagal S. Parsomnias in childhood. *Sleep Med Rev.* 2009;13:157-168.

National Institutes of Health. *NIH curriculum supplement series [Internet]: Information about sleep.* Bethesda, MD; 2007. Available at: http://www.ncbi.nlm.nih.gov/books/NBK20359/. Accessed June 10, 2015.

QUESTION 16

What Are Night Terrors?

Robert Heinle, MD

A piercing scream tears through the house in the middle of the night. There is screaming from the child's bedroom, parents come running to the bedside, and confusion and concern results. This is not an action sequence from a horror movie, but a unique parasomnia known as *night terrors*. As detailed in Question 7, parasomnias are undesirable physical events or experiences that occur during entry into sleep, within sleep, or during arousals from sleep. Parasomnias often have characteristics of both sleep and wakefulness, such as talking or movements, and often occur during transitions between sleep stages. Night terrors (also known as *sleep terrors*) are parasomnias that occur when a child has an atypical transition from slow-wave sleep to wakefulness. Because slow-wave sleep is a sleep stage within the broader category of non-rapid eye movement (NREM) sleep that occurs most frequently in the early part of the night, these episodes of night terrors typically happen in the first half of the night.

The typical night terror event is a dramatic and frightening episode (to the observer), in which a child appears to awaken suddenly a couple hours after falling asleep and becomes extremely agitated. These spells are usually initiated with a scream and the appearance of inconsolability. There is an autonomic surge of signals from the brain, leading to a fight-or-flight response with pupillary dilatation, flushing, sweating, and tachycardia. A look of fear will cover the face, but the child will only minimally interact with the environment, if he or she interacts at all. Most often, the child remains asleep, despite the dramatic nature of the episode and does not recall the event, even if he or she has been fully awakened by a frightened parent. Movements may be complex, including ambulation or even combative behavior, and there is a moderate risk for self-injury. Perception of the environment is altered and the child may behave in unexpected ways—even running into walls that were apparently unseen. The child is difficult to awaken and does not respond to soothing measures; in fact, soothing, touching, or stimulating the child may lead to increasing agitation. There is usually no recall of the event, although there may be a vague recollection of some threat, such as monsters, snakes, or spiders. A milder form may also be present as a nighttime awakening with feelings of dread, but without significant autonomic surge or agitation.

Chidekel AS, ed. *Curbside Consultation in Pediatric Sleep Disorders: 49 Clinical Questions* (pp. 73-75)

Table 16-1

Management of Night Terrors

- Reassure parents
  - No need to awaken child
  - Safety
  - Avoid secondary gain
- Phase shift
  - Afternoon nap to decrease Stage 3 sleep
  - Scheduled awakening at approximately 1 hour into sleep
- Medical management is rarely indicated
  - Benzodiazepines

Onset of night terrors is between 2 and 10 years of age, with a peak in the early school ages. Prevalence is reported at 3% to 4% in this age group, and the episodes typically decrease in frequency and severity over time. Although resolution usually occurs by adolescence, there are persistent episodes in some adults—typically less than 1% of all adults. There is a strong genetic predisposition to night terrors, and first-degree relatives of people with night terrors have a tenfold increase in incidence over the general population. If both parents were affected by night terrors, there is a 60% risk of night terrors in their children. In one case series, there was a 3-generational family with autosomal dominant inheritance pattern of night terrors. Exacerbating factors include sleep deprivation, illnesses, medications (eg, sedating hypnotics, stimulants, antihistamines), obstructive sleep apnea, periodic limb movements, and gastroesophageal reflux.

The differential diagnosis includes nightmares, nocturnal panic attacks, epileptic events, and cluster headaches. Nightmares do not typically involve significant ambulation, there is full recall of the nightmare, and, although initially agitated, children often respond quickly to reassuring and soothing measures. People with nocturnal panic attacks usually have a history of panic attacks during the day, are able to fully recall the panic attack, and are fully coherent during the event. Nocturnal seizures, particularly nocturnal frontal lobe epilepsy, may mimic night terrors; however, there is usually a history of seizures, the events occur at any time of night, and repeated events throughout the night are common and are usually associated with stereotypical movements. Cluster headaches typically occur with unilateral eye pain, with pupillary constriction, and in clusters.

Diagnosis is usually made by history and does not typically require testing such as polysomnogram unless the history is complex or atypical or suggests the additional presence of obstructive sleep apnea or periodic limb movements that may exacerbate night terrors. Exacerbating factors, such as sleep deprivation, should be avoided. Treating gastroesophageal reflux should be considered if clinical symptoms are present. Because of the moderate risk for self-injury, ensuring a safe environment is the mainstay of therapy. The sleep environment should be evaluated for corners, sharp objects, and access to stairs. Preemptive or scheduled awakenings are possible since episodes tend to occur around the same time of night; however, it remains somewhat controversial since waking may precipitate an event. Parents should be reassured of the benign nature and course of night terrors. Simple treatment options of night terrors are outlined in Table 16-1.

Summary

Night terrors are dramatic parasomnias with a typical presentation consistent with a fight-or-flight response leading to a clinical diagnosis. They may be associated with self-injury, and establishing a safe sleeping environment is imperative. Parents often require reassurance of the benign nature of night terrors and of the tendency toward self-resolution by adolescence.

Suggested Readings

American Academy of Sleep Medicine. *International Classification of Sleep Disorders: Diagnostic and Coding Manual*, 2nd ed. Westchester, IL: American Academy of Sleep Medicine; 2005.

Mason TBA, Pack AI. Pediatric parasomnias. *SLEEP.* 2007:30(2);141-151.

Avidan AY, Kaplish N. The parasomnias: epidemiologyclinical features, and diagnostic approach. *Clin Chest Med.* 2010;31:353-370.

Kotagal S. Parsomnias in childhood. *Sleep Med Rev.* 2009;13:157-168.

National Institutes of Health. *NIH curriculum supplement series [Internet]: Information about sleep.* Bethesda, MD; 2007. Available at: http://www.ncbi.nlm.nih.gov/books/NBK20359/. Accessed June 10, 2015.

QUESTION 17

WHAT IS BEHAVIORAL INSOMNIA OF CHILDHOOD?

Jennifer L. Curran, PhD and Jennifer Shroff Pendley, PhD

Behavioral sleep problems are very common in young children and can be very stressful for families. When one child is not sleeping, it is often the case that the entire household becomes sleep deprived. *The International Classification of Sleep Disorders, Second Edition*[1] describes 2 subtypes of behavioral insomnia of childhood—sleep onset association and limit-setting subtypes (Table 17-1). Both subtypes are described in more detail next.

Sleep Onset Association Subtype

Frequent or extended night awakenings is the typical presenting problem for children with behavioral insomnia of childhood, sleep onset association type. Sleep onset associations occur when certain conditions are necessary for a child to fall asleep. For example, a sleep association occurs when a child must suck his or her thumb or have her caregiver next to her in order to fall asleep. When these conditions are present at sleep onset, they usually must occur for the child to return to sleep during the night following normal arousals. Thus, if children associate their caregivers with sleep onset, when they awake during the night, they frequently are unable to fall back asleep on their own. Adults can relate to sleep associations in that, if their pillow falls on the ground during the night, they often cannot fall back asleep after a normal sleep cycle arousal without retrieving it.

That being said, some sleep onset associations are positive and should be encouraged. When children are able to self-soothe back to sleep, this would be considered a positive sleep onset association. For example, a child may use a blanket, pillow, stuffed animal, pacifier, or his or her thumb as strategies for self-soothing. However, when the child requires adult assistance with falling back to sleep, this would be considered a negative sleep association (eg, caregiver lying beside the child, riding in the car), as these rituals become disruptive for the whole household.

Chidekel AS, ed. *Curbside Consultation in Pediatric Sleep Disorders: 49 Clinical Questions* (pp. 77-80)

Table 17-1

Subtypes and Features of Behavioral Insomnia of Childhood

- Sleep onset association type
  - Certain conditions required for sleep onset
  - Sleep onset is a prolonged process without these conditions being met
  - Sleep onset conditions or associations are difficult and disruptive
  - Any nighttime awakenings require intervention to facilitate return to sleep
- Limit-setting type
  - Sleep onset is a difficult and prolonged process
  - Sleep onset is associated with bedtime resistance, refusal, and stalling
  - Sleep onset is associated with demands, requests, or curtain calls by the child
  - Inadequate parental or care giver limit-setting facilitates or prolongs this cycle
- Mixed type
  - Sleep onset is associated with elements of both the need for associations or conditions, as well as bedtime resistance, refusal, or stalling that is inadequately addressed by the parent or caregiver

Adapted from American Academy of Sleep Medicine. *International Classification of Sleep Disorders, 2nd ed: Diagnostic and Coding Manual.* Westchester, IL: American Academy of Sleep Medicine; 2005.

The ability to self-soothe is a developmental skill that can play a role in sleep behaviors and positive sleep associations. Self-soothing at sleep onset and following nighttime awakenings develops between 3 and 6 months of age and is typically accomplished by 12 months.[2] For this reason, a diagnosis of behavioral sleep insomnia, sleep onset association type, is not considered appropriate before 6 months of age.[3]

Limit-Setting Subtype

Sleep problems resulting from difficulties with enforcing bedtime limits generally fall within the category of behavioral insomnia of childhood, limit-setting type. These sleep difficulties typically begin during the toddler years, when children move out of their cribs and can leave their room. Toddlers may try to stall bedtime by begging to watch additional television, pleading to read another story, requesting numerous drinks or snacks, and asking to use the bathroom. Children may also outright refuse to go to bed by refusing to do tasks associated with the bedtime routine (eg, get pajamas on, brush teeth, go to room) and/or refusing to remain in bed by following the caregiver back to other rooms of the house or playing in his or her room. Other behaviors that are

Table 17-2

General Treatment Principles of Behavioral Insomnia of Childhood

Establish sleep hygiene • Bedtime routine • Promote self-soothing Behavioral techniques • Extinction • Graduated extinction • Bedtime fading	Limit setting • Consistent reinforcement

typical with limit-setting challenges include children falling asleep while watching television and falling asleep in a room other than their own.

These problematic sleep behaviors, whether stalling or refusing, start because they elicit a response from caregivers. Over time, children learn that asking to go to the bathroom or refusing to get in bed, for example, result in delaying their bedtime and/or allowing them to engage in a preferred activity (eg, watching television).

In clinical practice, it is not uncommon to encounter elements of both types of behavioral insomnia of childhood in a single patient. A detailed sleep history and discussion of both bedtime and nighttime sleep problems can identify all of the aspects of a child's sleep problems so that a treatment plan can be devised and established.

Treatment

Bedtime problems and night waking in children often do not resolve on their own. If left untreated, behavioral insomnia can lead to increased irritability, temper tantrums, and behavior difficulties, as well as sleep deprivation for the entire family. Behavioral strategies are discussed in Question 14 and the establishment of sleep hygiene will be discussed in Question 18. The treatment of behavioral insomnia is briefly outlined in Table 17-2. Sleep specialists or other professionals who specialize in behavior management can be helpful in providing suggestions to minimize these difficulties. See the "Suggested Readings" section at the end of this chapter for helpful resources for caregivers.

References

1. American Academy of Sleep Medicine. *International Classification of Sleep Disorders, 2nd ed.: Diagnostic and Coding Manual.* Westchester, IL: American Academy of Sleep Medicine; 2005.
2. Goodlin-Jones BL, Burnham MM, Gaylor EE, Anders TF. Night waking, sleep-wake organization, and self soothing in the first year of life. *JDBP.* 2001;22:226-233.
3. Meltzer LJ. Clinical management of behavioral insomnia of childhood: treatment of bedtime problems and night waking in young children. *Behav Sleep Med.* 2010;8:172-189.

Suggested Readings

Ferber, R. *Solve Your Child's Sleep Problems.* New York: Fireside; 2006.

Mindell JA. *Sleeping Through the Night, Revised Edition: How Infants, Toddlers, and Their Parents Can Get a Good Night's Sleep.* New York: HarperCollins Publishers; 2005.

Owens, JA, Mindell JA. *Take Charge of Your Child's Sleep: The All-in-One Resource for Solving Sleep Problems in Kids and Teens.* New York: Marlow & Company; 2005.

QUESTION 18

What Are Some Pearls or Strategies to Manage or, Even Better, to Prevent Behavioral Sleep Disorders in Young Children?

Meghan McAuliffe Lines, PhD and Cheyenne Hughes-Reid, PhD

Adequate sleep is critical for children's health, and the establishment of positive sleep associations and routines is essential to preventing sleep difficulties. Bedtime problems are a common concern in young children, occurring in 20% to 30% of infants, toddlers, and preschoolers.[1] The most common sleep problems that occur in childhood are related to sleep onset, sleep resistance, or night awakenings. There are evidence-based recommendations for the prevention and management of sleep problems in children. Given the critical role of sleep in children's healthy development, pediatricians should routinely assess sleep and provide parents with anticipatory guidance at well-child visits.[2,3]

There is a bidirectional relationship between sleep problems and mood and behavior disorders in children. Children with mood and behavior disorders often experience sleep problems, and sleep deprivation can also result in display or exacerbation of mood and behavior symptoms. It is important for clinicians to recognize this relationship and assess for sleep concerns in children presenting with behavioral issues, and vice versa (Figure 18-1).[4]

Chidekel AS, ed. *Curbside Consultation in Pediatric Sleep Disorders: 49 Clinical Questions* (pp. 81-85)

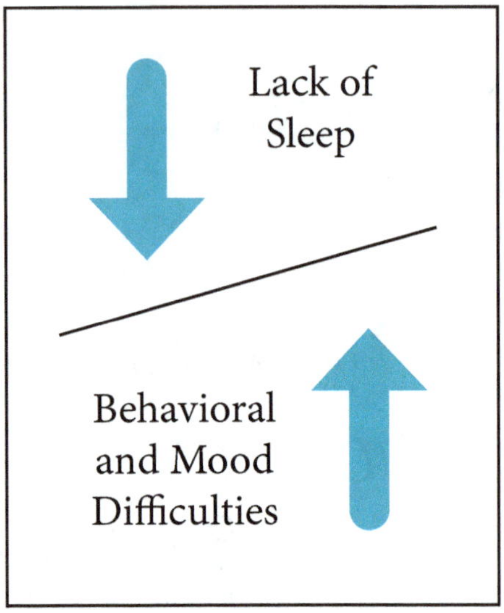

Figure 18-1. Bidirectional relationship between sleep and mood and behavior difficulties.

Prevention of Sleep Problems

Sleep Hygiene

Sleep hygiene strategies are daily practices that set the stage for healthy sleep. The acronym SLEEPS can help clinicians recall the components of good sleep hygiene for young children, which include the following[4]:

- Schedule: A sleep schedule, including a set bedtime, consistent morning wake times, and age-appropriate naps, should be followed. Long and/or frequent naps may interfere with nighttime sleep and should be avoided.
- Light snack: A light snack before bed may help with sleep onset. Heavy meals and foods or beverages containing caffeine should be avoided.
- Environment: Make sure the child's room is comfortable—cool, dark, and quiet.
- Established routine: A routine that consists of 3 to 4 calming, enjoyable activities should be established. Examples of activities include taking a bath, reading a book, and listening to soft music or lullabies.
- Physical activity: Daily physical activity can be helpful for sleep onset and sleep quality. Physical activity in the hour before bedtime should be avoided.
- Soothing activities: For at least 1 hour before bedtime, activities should be limited to quiet and calming activities. Stimulating activities such as outdoor play, television, and video games should be avoided.

Sleep Associations

Children associate the conditions that are present at bedtime with falling asleep. If these conditions include a caregiver (eg, rocking, rubbing their back, laying down with them) or a different location (eg, parent's bed, sofa), then children often have difficulty getting back to sleep independently when they wake during the night.[5] It is critical for children to lay in their own bed alone when drowsy in order to make the proper associations with sleep. Transitional objects, such as a blanket or favorite stuffed animal, may aid in independent sleep.

Behavioral Reinforcement

Praise and positive attention for behaviors that are consistent with sleep can help children to establish good sleep behaviors. Caregivers can help by providing children with attention for sleep-compatible behaviors, such as putting on their pajamas or getting into bed. Behaviors that are not compatible with sleep should be ignored.

Management of Sleep Problems

Graduated Extinction

The graduated extinction method is designed to help children learn the self-soothing skills required for falling asleep independently.[1,4,6] In this method (discussed in greater detail in Question 14), after the completion of the bedtime routine, the caregiver leaves the room while the child is still awake, but then checks in briefly at specified intervals. During check-ins, the caregiver briefly reassures the child, and then leaves the room until the next check-in. If desired, the interval between check-ins can gradually be increased.

Bedtime Pass

The bedtime pass is an intervention also based on extinction and is ideal for young children who frequently make requests for another story, another drink, or an extra hug before bed.[7,8] The child is provided a "pass" that may be redeemed for one caregiver visit after bedtime. The caregiver should ignore all other requests from the child and respond only to the one pass.

Bedtime Fading

An alternative strategy for getting a child to go to sleep at night while minimizing conflict is to keep them up later than their typical bedtime. In bedtime fading, the child's bedtime is delayed to ensure sleep initiation with minimal resistance. Once the child is able to fall asleep quickly at the later time, then bedtime can be moved earlier by 15 to 30 minutes per night until the desired bedtime is achieved.[1,6]

Behavioral Reinforcement

Behavioral reinforcement systems, such as sticker charts, can be particularly effective with helping preschool children to adopt new behaviors.[4] As with any reward system, the greatest success will be achieved when clear goals are established and rewards are provided immediately. Over time, goals should be increased and the frequency of reward should be decreased. If desired, a behavioral reinforcement system can be paired with the bedtime pass. In this instance, the child could receive a reward in the morning if the bedtime pass was not used during the night.

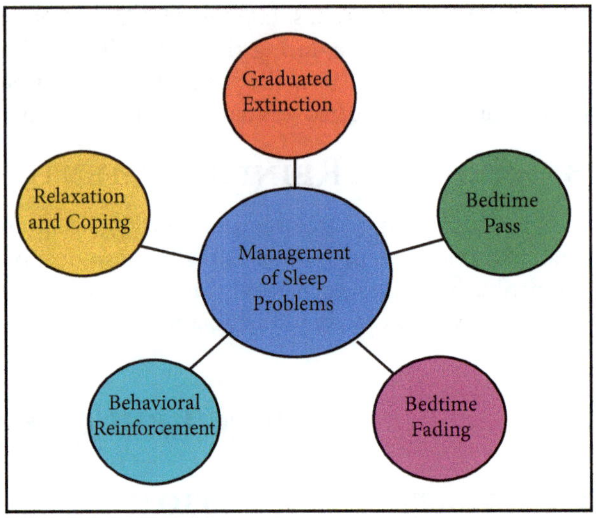

Figure 18-2. Strategies for the management of sleep problems in children.

Relaxation and Coping

Relaxation strategies and coping statements may be an effective method when nighttime fears are contributing the sleep problems.[2] Possible relaxation strategies include deep breathing, muscle relaxation, and imagery. In addition to using these relaxation techniques, children can be taught to use positive coping statements, such as "I can take care of myself in my bed at night" (Figure 18-2).

Summary

Sleep difficulties are often overlooked and can be related to a host of other health and behavioral concerns. Independent sleep is one of the most important gifts that caregivers can provide to their child. Given the prevalence rate of sleep problems in young children, pediatricians can play a key role in assessing sleep, providing parents with anticipatory guidance regarding healthy sleep development and offering strategies to manage sleep concerns. Pediatricians are encouraged to address these issues at each well-child visit, as well as to explore issues related to sleep when additional health and behavior concerns arise.

References

1. Mindell JA, Kuhn B, Lewis, DS, et al. Behavioral treatment of bedtime problems and night wakings in infants and young children. *Sleep*. 2006;29(10):1263-1276.
2. Christophersen ER, Mortweet SL. *Treatments That Work With Children: Empirically Supported Strategies for Managing Childhood Problems*. Washington, DC: American Psychological Association; 2001.
3. Hagan JF, Shaw JS, Duncan, PM, eds. *Bright Futures: Guidelines for Health Supervision of Infants, Children, and Adolescents, Third Edition*. Elk Grove Village: American Academy of Pediatrics; 2008.
4. Mindell JA, Owens JD. *A Clinical Guide to Pediatric Sleep: Diagnosis and Management of Sleep Problems*. Philadelphia: Wolters Kluwer Health/Lippincott Williams & Wilkins; 2009.
5. Ferber R. *Solve Your Child's Sleep Problems*. London, UK: Ebury Publishing; 2013.

6. Durand VM. *Sleep Better! A Guide to Improving Sleep for Children With Special Needs*. Baltimore, MD: Paul H. Brookes Publishing Company; 1998.
7. Freeman KA. Treating bedtime resistance with the bedtime pass: a systematic replication and component analysis with 3-year-olds. *J Appl Behav Anal.* 2006;39(4):423.
8. Moore BA, Friman PC, Fruzzetti AE et al. Brief report: evaluating the bedtime pass program for child resistance to bedtime—a randomized, controlled trial. *J Pediatr Psychol.* 2007;32(3)283-287.

SECTION IV

SLEEP ISSUES THAT ARE UNIQUE TO ADOLESCENTS

QUESTION 19

Some of My Teenage Patients Are Staying Up Late and Then Having Difficulty Getting Up for School. Do They Have Insomnia?

Johanna Carpenter, PhD and Kari Baber, PhD

Adolescents have different sleep patterns than both younger children and adults. In general, adolescents sleep for longer on weekends than weekdays, sleep for fewer hours on weeknights than they did as younger children, and typically take longer than children to fall asleep.[1] Behavioral and environmental factors (eg, less parental control over bedtime, more time spent on homework and extracurricular activities after school) are often cited as reasons for changes in adolescent sleep patterns. However, adolescents also demonstrate changes in circadian rhythms and physiological sleep regulation patterns. Specifically, compared to adults, adolescents tend to experience longer periods of active, alert wakefulness that occur later in the day.[1] Therefore, for many adolescent patients, staying up late and then having difficulty awakening in time for school may reflect normal shifts in sleep patterns. Although adolescent patients may naturally gravitate toward sleeping and staying up later than they did as younger children, complaints from patients (or, more often, parents) about sleep patterns warrant further discussion.

We discuss 2 types of sleep disorders that could be involved when adolescents are reporting late bedtimes and difficulty waking up: pediatric insomnia and delayed sleep phase disorder. However, for 2 reasons, it is important not to place too much emphasis on these diagnoses. First, adolescents can exhibit impaired daytime functioning and require intervention even if their sleep difficulties are subclinical in nature or seem related to normative sleep schedule shifts. Second, there can be myriad reasons why adolescents are staying up late and not getting enough sleep. These reasons are important to understand because they are likely to shape the type and content of intervention that is recommended to the patient. Therefore, we also provide questions that aim to help differentiate between various issues that could be underlying sleep difficulties, such as the following:

- Mental health concerns
- Lifestyle issues
- Sleep hygiene issues

Chidekel AS, ed. *Curbside Consultation in Pediatric Sleep Disorders: 49 Clinical Questions* (pp. 89-92)

Finally, we provide suggestions to help pediatricians determine whether to provide a referral for patients with sleep disturbances or to manage sleep concerns in the primary care office.

Insomnia

As many as 25% of adolescents may experience symptoms of insomnia, with relatively fewer of them (approximately 5%) meeting diagnostic criteria for a diagnosis of pediatric insomnia.[2] Pediatric insomnia can refer to transient or chronic difficulty with sleep initiation, duration, consolidation, or quality that occurs despite age-appropriate time and opportunity for sleep, resulting in daytime functional impairment for the child and/or family. In order to be considered a disorder, insomnia cannot be occurring secondary to another sleep disturbance or a psychiatric or medical problem. A short-term course of insomnia may be related to experiencing a stressful event or transition. Importantly, this definition of insomnia recognizes that expected times and opportunities for sleep vary with age.

Delayed Sleep Phase Disorder (Circadian Rhythm Disorder)

Adolescents whose sleep-wake schedule is significantly and persistently delayed (by at least 2 hours beyond the desired bedtime) may meet diagnostic criteria for delayed sleep phase disorder (DSPD) or, as it is now known, *circadian rhythm disorder, delayed sleep phase type*. Prevalence estimates range from below 1% among adolescents in the general population to 10% of patients with insomnia complaints in sleep clinics.[1] Adolescents with DSPD frequently report falling asleep in the early morning hours and experiencing significant difficulty awakening in the morning to attend school or work. When patients attempt to follow a conventional sleep schedule, they experience insomnia, daytime sleepiness, and functional impairment. When sleeping according to the delayed schedule, however, sleep latency, duration, and quality are normal. In this way, DSPD can be differentiated from insomnia, which involves difficulty falling or staying asleep, regardless of bedtime. Adolescents with DSPD experience insomnia only when they are attempting to follow a conventional schedule with a much earlier bedtime.[3] DSPD also must be differentiated from normal adolescent sleep patterns, which would be characterized by a delayed schedule in the absence of distress or functional impairment.[1]

Assessing Contributing Factors to the Sleep Disturbance

Adolescent patients can present with similar complaints of sleep disturbance, but very different associated or contributing factors. In assessing sleep difficulties, pediatricians should screen for mental health concerns, lifestyle issues, and/or sleep hygiene issues that could be contributing to sleep difficulties. Careful assessment is important in order to refer patients out to appropriate providers (eg, mental health provider vs sleep medicine physician) and to identify sleep-related goals and intervention targets.

Mental Health Concerns

Mental health concerns can be both a cause and consequence of sleep difficulties.[3] Specifically, difficulty sleeping has been associated with attention problems, anxiety, depression, and social withdrawal. In adolescence, symptoms of mood/anxiety disorders may be particularly important to assess. The following questions may be helpful to ask adolescents and/or their caregivers:

- Do you have difficulty falling asleep because you are worrying or planning for the next day?
- Do you have frequent aches and pains (unrelated to known medical illness)?
- Is there anything you have been worrying about lately?
- Is it hard to "turn off" your brain at night?
- Are you feeling sad, upset, or grouchier than usual?
- Have you recently experienced a significant stressor, or are you anticipating an upcoming event?
- Are you still enjoying activities that used to be fun for you?
- How are you feeling about how things in your life are going?

Lifestyle Issues

Late-night activities may delay bedtime beyond the desired time and result in difficulty awakening, particularly for adolescents who are overscheduled during the after-school hours or demonstrate poor time management skills that delay schoolwork. Symptoms of insomnia or delayed sleep phase may not be present, but adolescents may perceive a lack of opportunity to sleep more. Questions such as the following may be helpful:

- Are you staying up late in order to talk to friends, use social media, complete homework, and/or study for tests?
- Do you have after-school, work, leisure, and/or household responsibilities that delay homework completion and/or bedtime?
- Would you be able to go to bed earlier and sleep more if you were not doing other things?

Sleep Hygiene Issues

Good sleep practices are prerequisites for the development of adaptive sleep routines in adolescence. Sleep concerns, particularly complaints of insomnia, are often associated with poor sleep hygiene. The following questions may be helpful to determine if sleep hygiene issues are contributing to adolescent sleep concerns:

- Do you have a bedtime routine? What is it?
- Do you take any medications or herbal supplements?
- Do you exercise? When?
- How often do you take daytime or evening naps? When, and for how long?
- When is your last meal before bedtime?

- What electronics do you have in your bedroom?
- Do you ever do homework, watch television, or use other electronic devices in bed?
- Do you consume caffeine in the afternoon or evening?
- Is your room dark enough, quiet enough, and the right temperature for you to sleep?

When to Manage vs Refer Out for the Treatment of Adolescent Sleep Problems

A referral to a sleep center or sleep medicine physician should be considered when an additional physiological sleep disorder is suspected (eg, sleep apnea) or when sleep problems do not respond to intervention, cause significant functional impairment, and/or are occurring in the context of other special developmental or medical needs. Also, because behavioral treatments for insomnia or DSPD often require specialized knowledge of behavioral sleep medicine, these concerns may be best treated by, or treated in close consultation with, a sleep specialist. Treatment for DSPD can involve shifting sleep timing using behavioral and/or pharmacological approaches (including melatonin). Treatment for insomnia may include sleep opportunity restriction (ie, limiting time in bed to total sleep time), relaxation strategies, and cognitive reframing.[3] It also is recommended that a referral for mental health services be provided for patients who are presenting with a comorbid psychiatric concern, such as depressed mood, anxiety, or anger.

Pediatricians may choose to manage other sleep concerns in the primary care office (eg, those that are primarily sleep hygiene-related or lifestyle-related). A 2-week sleep diary is recommended to gain an accurate snapshot of the patient's sleep profile and to help evaluate progress (a free 2-week sleep diary is available from the American Academy of Sleep Medicine[4]). Interventions may include problem-solving with adolescent patients and family members about, for example, establishing a bedtime routine, restructuring or rearranging home activities, removing electronic devices from the bedroom, prioritizing homework completion before leisure activities, and/or limiting or eliminating caffeinated beverages. Any goals set with families should be manageable, specific, and measurable. If adolescents are resistant to making changes, it can be helpful to implement short-term behavioral agreements with reasonable incentives for following a sleep plan.

References

1. Crowley SJ, Acebo C, Carskadon MA. Sleep, circadian rhythms, and delayed phase in adolescents. *Sleep Med.* 2007;8:602-612.
2. Roberts RE, Roberts CR, Duong HT. Chronic insomnia and its negative consequences for health and functioning of adolescents: a 12-month prospective study. *J Adolesc Health.* 2008;42:294-302.
3. Mindell JA, Meltzer LJ. Behavioural sleep disorders in children and adolescents. *Ann Acad Med Singapore.* 2008;37:722-728.
4. American Academy of Sleep Medicine. *Two week sleep diary.* Available at www.yoursleep.aasmnet.org/pdf/sleepdiary.pdf. Accessed 2/28/13.

QUESTION 20

Some of My Teenage Patients Complain of Being Tired All the Time. When Do I Need to Be Concerned?

Christina Calamaro, PhD, CRNP

Consistent and sufficient sleep allows for optimal cognition, emotion, and success at performance-related functions. Insufficient sleep exacerbates multiple comorbid conditions and can lead to harmful, even life-threatening, sequelae. Excessive sleepiness is also associated with reduced short-term memory and learning ability, negative mood, inconsistent performance, poor productivity, and loss of some forms of behavioral control. Adolescents and young adults (ages 12 to 25 years) are a population at high risk for problems that are sleepiness-based and it is well documented that adolescents often shortchange their need for sleep and attempt to function on a regular basis, with less than the recommended sleep hours each day. To provide recommendations for adolescent sleep, it is important to understand pubertal effects, changes in sleep patterns and consequences of daytime sleepiness, and environmental influences on adolescent sleep patterns and sleep duration. Also, the impact of sleeplessness on mental health and disease states will be reviewed.

Pubertal Effects of Sleep

Several changes in sleep patterns, sleep-wake cycling, and circadian timing systems are associated with puberty, which is also a time of both physiological and social changes that affect sleep. With the onset of puberty, most adolescents begin to experience a sleep-wake "phase delay." This phase delay manifests as a phase delay of the sleep-wake cycle of up to 2 hours, starting with pubertal onset. Two biological changes are the principal causes of this change in sleep regulation. First, during puberty, delayed secretion of melatonin has been demonstrated; this delay, in concert

Chidekel AS, ed. *Curbside Consultation in Pediatric Sleep Disorders: 49 Clinical Questions* (pp. 93-95)

with a parallel shift in circadian phase to an evening preference from a morning preference, results in difficulty for the adolescent to fall asleep at an early bedtime. The second biological factor is an altered sleep drive (Process S), resulting in a slower accumulation of pressure to fall asleep. This is demonstrated by the adolescent brain's response to sleep loss and by a longer time to fall asleep after being awake for approximately 14.5 to 18.5 hours in post- vs pre-adolescents. As a child moves through puberty, these factors provide the impetus for the adolescent to stay awake for longer and later hours. Contrasting this is evidence from multiple studies that adolescent sleep needs do not decline from pre-adolescent levels, with an optimal sleep time for this age group of at least 7.5 to 9 hours. There is individual variability with sleep needs and timing, but research has indicated that the average adolescent has difficulty falling asleep before 11:00 p.m. and is best suited to awaken at 8:00 a.m. or later.

Daytime Sleepiness in Adolescents

Adolescents and young adults (aged 12 to 25 years) are a population at high risk for problem sleepiness. In fact, it is well documented that adolescents often shortchange their need for sleep and attempt to function on a regular basis with fewer than the recommended sleep hours each day. The resultant excessive sleepiness has a negative impact on daytime functioning in adolescents, increasing their risk of injury and death. Drowsiness or fatigue has been identified as a principal cause in 100,000 or more traffic crashes each year. Insufficient sleep also takes a toll on academics. In a recent National Sleep Foundation poll, 20% to 28% of students reported falling asleep in school at least once per week, and more than 1 in 5 fell asleep doing homework. Many studies also show an association between insufficient sleep and lower academic achievement at middle, high school, and collegiate levels. Finally, insufficient sleep has been associated with higher rates of absenteeism, tardiness, and decreased readiness to learn.

Sleep restriction has effects on multiple disease processes. Obesity, asthma, eczema, diabetes, and obstructive sleep apnea have all been further exacerbated by insufficient sleep in adolescents. Mental health issues are significantly worsened in the presence of insufficient sleep. Studies have reported greater depressed mood in those adolescents who went to sleep on the weekend 2 or more hours later than their typical weeknight bedtime, as compared to those who did not stay up late on the weekends. Studies also suggest that sleep loss may be associated with a decreased ability to control, inhibit, or change emotional responses. Also concerning are studies that report strong associations of shorter sleep times with conduct and aggressive behaviors, impulsivity, problems completing tasks, and inability to stay on task.

Given this, it is important to understand the risk factors that impact sleep duration in this population. With the pubertal drive to stay awake, and desire to maintain constant contact with their social network through increasing technology use, adolescents turn to higher doses of stimulants, such as caffeine or nicotine, to stay awake. More than 80% of adolescents sleep with cell phones or have them within reach, leading to potential sleep disruption. Adolescents frequently have multiple technologies in the bedroom, leading to greater potential for sleep disruption and insufficient sleep. Inappropriate stimulant use and access to multiple technologies in the bedroom, combined with early school start times, have created a population of students at risk for significant health risk from insufficient sleep.

Table 20-1

Elements of Adolescent Sleep Hygiene

- Allow adequate time for sleep.
- Avoid stimulant use after lunch time.
- Eliminate or minimize technology use 1 to 2 hours before bedtime.
- Make the bedroom a technology-free zone when it is time to sleep.
- Maintain a regular and reasonable bedtime with parental input and monitoring.
- Use morning light to promote wakefulness and reinforce circadian timing.

Improving Adolescent Sleep

It is important to set goals with adolescents to help them understand the need to establish healthy sleep routines that may last a lifetime (Table 20-1). These habits include several key elements. It is important that they sleep 8 to 10 hours each night; avoid caffeine and other stimulants late in the day (preferably having none of these after 12 p.m.); gain exposure to bright light in the morning to reinforce the brain's circadian timing system; and shut down technology at least 1 to 2 hours before bedtime to allow the body to relax and create an environment conducive to quality sleep (most importantly, this includes keeping the cell phone and other portable technology out of the bedroom when it is time for sleep). Several school districts and systems are changing the timing of school schedules and related activities to accommodate adolescents' sleep needs and behaviors. Adolescent students, because of circadian rhythm timing, are most likely to be alert and be able to learn with later school times and later high school schedules.

Suggested Readings

American Academy of Pediatrics, Adolescent Sleep Working Group, Committee on Adolescence, Council on School Health. School start times for adolescents. *Pediatrics*. 2014;134(3):642-649.

Calamaro, CJ, Mason, TA, Ratcliffe, SJ. Adolescents living the 24/7 lifestyle: effects of caffeine and technology on sleep duration and daytime functioning. *Pediatrics.* 2009;123(6):e1005-e1010.

Carskadon, MA. Sleep in adolescents: the perfect storm. *Pediatr Clin North Am.* 2011;58(3):637-647.

Carskadon MA, Wolfson AR, Acebo C, Tzischinsky O, Seifer R. Adolescent sleep patterns, circadian timing, and sleepiness at a transition to early school days. *SLEEP.* 1998;21:871-881.

Dahl RE. The impact of inadequate sleep on children's daytime cognitive function. *Semin Pediatr Neurol.* 1996; 3(1):44-50.

National Sleep Foundation. *Teens and sleep.* http://sleepfoundation.org/sleep-topics/teens-and-sleep. Accessed March 15, 2015.

Owens, J. Adolescent Sleep Working Group and Committee on Adolescence. Insufficient sleep in adolescents and young adults: an update on causes and consequences. *Pediatrics*. 2014;134(3):e921-e932.

Wolfson AR, Carskadon MA. Sleep schedules and daytime functioning in adolescents. *Child Development.* 1998;69:875-887.

21

QUESTION

Is Sleep Deprivation Really That Big of a Problem in Adolescents?

Holger Link, MD

Sleep deprivation in adolescents is a significant and growing problem. Most adolescents in the United States are not getting enough sleep. A 2011 survey by the National Sleep Foundation found that 6 out of 10 teenagers are getting fewer than 8 hours of sleep per night and are waking up in the morning feeling unrefreshed at least a few days per week. Even more disturbing is the finding that 4 out of 10 teenagers have driven a car while feeling drowsy. Teenagers are the least experienced drivers, are more easily distracted by their peers when driving, and are at high risk for sleepiness-related accidents.

The optimal sleep duration for most adolescents is somewhere between 8 to 10 hours of sleep per night. In reality, most do not meet this goal and the average sleep duration deviates further down from these recommendations as children move from early to late adolescence. There are also significant differences in sleep duration across the world. Teenagers in Europe sleep the longest, while teenagers in the United States are somewhere in the middle, and teenagers from Asia have the shortest sleep duration (40 to 60 minutes less each night than their American counterparts). The specific reasons for these differences in sleep duration are unknown. Defining the optimal sleep duration is further complicated by the fact that teenagers have different sleep needs depending on their genetic predisposition, their overall health, and the physical and cognitive demands placed on them during the daytime.

Most adolescents suffer from acute and chronic sleep deprivation. Chronic sleep deprivation, like the debt on a credit card, accumulates over time and, depending on how much a teenager's sleep time falls short each day, it can reach clinical significance either fairly rapidly over a few weeks or slowly over the course of a few months. A teenager that is consistently getting just 30 to 60 minutes less sleep than he or she biologically requires can accrue a clinically significant sleep deficit. The good news is that sleep debt does not need to be paid off hour by hour. A teenager can significantly reduce an existing large sleep debt with as few as 3 to 4 nights of 9 to 10 hours of sleep, with resultant improvements in daytime functioning.

Chidekel AS, ed. *Curbside Consultation in Pediatric Sleep Disorders: 49 Clinical Questions* (pp. 97-99)

There are a number of factors that contribute to sleep deprivation in adolescents. Many teenagers have a demanding schedule and are trying to fit school, homework, sports, and social activities into an ever-shrinking day. It is also close to impossible to find a teenager nowadays who does not have a smart phone or a computer in the bedroom. Given their packed schedules, a majority of teenagers use the time before falling asleep to catch up with their peers, play games, or listen to music on their electronic devices. A considerable number of teens sleep with the phone on active ringer in their bedroom.

In addition to these external forces, important changes are taking place within the circadian system during adolescence. The internal body clock naturally drifts to a later time as children enter adolescence. This, in turn, delays the time at which the body and brain are ready to fall asleep. Unfortunately, school start times are earlier or at the same time, but rarely later, as teenagers enter high school. This combination of later bedtime and earlier school start times can fairly quickly lead to a significant sleep deficit. Furthermore, some adolescents will develop a more severe delay in circadian rhythm that is known as *delayed sleep phase syndrome*. These individuals cannot fall asleep at an appropriate time, have a very difficult time waking up in the morning, and quickly accumulate a sleep deficit that interferes with their daytime functioning.

Teenagers are going through dramatic hormonal, physical, and emotional changes during adolescence. Sleep deprivation during this period of vulnerability has a strong potential to increase the possibility for reduced academic performance, school failure, risk-taking behaviors, mood disorders, and substance use. As more adolescents are feeling stressed, chronically fatigued, and sleepy, they are increasingly turning to alcohol, caffeine, and other drugs for help. Stimulant drugs like methylphenidate are being consumed at rising rates by high school and college students. They can relieve and mask the chronic sleepiness associated with sleep deprivation and are being used by students to improve endurance for studying and concentration during tests. While stimulant drugs help mitigate some of the effects of sleep deprivation, they do carry the risk for serious side effects and cannot replace adequate sleep. Furthermore, it is concerning that stimulant drugs are not always obtained through a prescribing physician, but increasingly through other students or friends. The unsupervised use of stimulant drugs increases the risk for physical and mental harm.

Another frequently used alerting drug is caffeine, which has historically been consumed in the form of coffee. More recently though, the source of caffeine has shifted to caffeinated energy drinks, some of which contain many times the dose of caffeine found in a cup of coffee. The increasing consumption of highly caffeinated energy drinks has raised concerns for life-threatening side effects because of overdosing and coingestion of alcohol. Even when not consumed in toxic doses, caffeine can have negative side effects. The sleep-inhibiting effects of caffeine and its relatively long half-life can further aggravate the problem of sleep deprivation as it will make it harder for the adolescent to fall asleep at an appropriate time. It is important to note that, while caffeine does have alerting effects, it does not replace adequate sleep.

Chronic sleep deprivation not only affects the brain, but has also been associated with negative hormonal and metabolic changes, increased inflammation, and increased risk for cardiovascular disease. Evidence is accumulating that shorter sleep duration is an independent risk factor for obesity. These negative effects of sleep deprivation are especially concerning given the obesity epidemic in the United States whereby now more than one-third of adolescents are overweight or obese. Clinical symptoms of sleep deprivation and potential questions that can be used to query patients and families are given in Table 21-1.

So what is a teenager to do in order to avoid getting hurt because of sleep deprivation? The best prevention is to get more sleep. This is often much easier said than done. Once the teenager has established unhealthy sleep habits, it is very hard to break them. Therefore, parents should start early and establish a bedroom environment for their pre-adolescent that is free from electronic devices. It is much harder to take a TV or computer away from a child than it is to avoid putting one in the bedroom in the first place. Parents should try to lead by example and make adequate

Table 21-1

An Overview of Sleep Deprivation in Adolescents

Symptoms of Sleep Deprivation

- Fatigue
- Mood changes
- Illness
- School tardiness
- Declining academic performance
- Falling asleep in school
- Sleepy driver accidents or fatalities

Clinical Questions

- Does your child need to be awakened for school?
- Does your child sleep 2 hours or more on weekends and vacations?
- Does your child fall asleep at inappropriate times?
- Does your child's behavior and mood differ after getting adequate sleep?

sleep a family priority. Naps after school can help, but longer naps can make it harder to go to bed at the appropriate time. Sleeping in on the weekends helps pay some of the sleep debt, but also risks further pushing the adolescent's body clock to a later bedtime. Bright light in the morning can help prevent a delay in the body clock. Conversely, light exposure in the evening will delay the body clock and make it harder to fall asleep at an appropriate time.

Summary

Sleep deprivation is a serious problem in adolescents with significant consequences. The forces that drive sleep deprivation in adolescents are likely to grow. Prevention is critical as it is difficult to reverse established unhealthy sleep habits.

Suggested Readings

Calamaro CJ, Mason TB, Ratcliffe SJ. Adolescents living the 24/7 lifestyle: effects of caffeine and technology on sleep duration and daytime functioning. *Pediatrics.* 2009;123(6):e1005-e1010.

Faraut B, Boudjeltia KZ, Vanhamme L, Kerkhofs M. Immune, inflammatory and cardiovascular consequences of sleep restriction and recovery. *Sleep Med Rev.* 2012;16(2):137-149.

Matricciani L, Blunden S, Rigney G, Williams MT, Olds TS. Children's sleep needs: is there sufficient evidence to recommend optimal sleep for children? *Sleep.* 2013;36(4):527-534.

Saxvig IW, Pallesen S, Wilhelmsen-Langeland A, Molde H, Bjorvatn B. Prevalence and correlates of delayed sleep phase in high school students. *Sleep Medicine.* 2012;13:193-199.

Taylor DJ, Bramoweth AD. Patterns and consequences of inadequate sleep in college students: substance use and motor vehicle accidents. *J Adolesc Health.* 2010;46(6):610-612.

Wolk BJ, Ganetsky M, Babu KM. Toxicity of energy drinks. *Curr Opin Pediatr.* 2012;24(2):243-251.

QUESTION 22

How Big of a Problem Is Drowsy Driving in Teen Drivers?

Holger Link, MD

Teenagers who are driving drowsy do not just have a big problem—they have a life and death problem. At no other time in a person's life will the risk for a fatal car crash be higher than during the teenage years. The absolute number of deaths due to a fatal car accident is twice as high in teenagers compared to any other age group. The National Highway Traffic Safety Administration performed an analysis of mortality among teenagers, looking at the time period from 1999 to 2006. Around 16,000 teenagers died per year during that time period. The death rate increased dramatically in teenagers over the age of 15 and the single most common cause of death was a fatal motor vehicle accident, followed by homicide, suicide, cancer, and heart disease. There are no precise data on near-miss events or nonfatal accidents, but it is likely that the fatalities only represent a small portion of the true impact of driving-related accidents.

The vast majority of teenager motor vehicle crashes are due to driver errors and not environmental or technical car problems. Multiple variables contribute to these errors and it is estimated that drowsiness is a major factor in about one-fifth of all motor vehicle crashes in the United States.

Many people in our society are chronically sleep-deprived, and teenagers are no exception. Unfortunately, the severity of sleep deprivation has been increasing over the past decades due to increased demands placed on teenagers from school and related activities, extracurricular activities, hobbies, the introduction of electronic entertainment into the bedroom, and the aggressive marketing of caffeine-containing energy drinks to teenagers. Poor sleep hygiene, insufficient sleep, and poor sleep quality are extremely common among teenagers nowadays. This increases their risk for clinically significant drowsiness, with resulting impairments in mood and behavior, learning, judgment, and driving performance.

Further complicating the issue is a lack of awareness in our society of the impact of drowsy driving on people's lives. Most people will agree that driving while under the influence of alcohol should be illegal. On the other hand, driving while drowsy does not appear to carry the same

Chidekel AS, ed. *Curbside Consultation in Pediatric Sleep Disorders: 49 Clinical Questions* (pp. 101-103)

stigma and level of concern. However, sleep deprivation and drowsiness impair judgment similar to the way that alcohol does.

Drowsy drivers can fall asleep repeatedly for a few seconds with complete lapses in consciousness without even being aware of it before, during, or after the episodes. This phenomenon is known as *microsleep* and it carries profound risks. A driver going 60 miles per hour will cover the length of a football field in just 4 seconds. Many bad and potentially fatal incidents can happen during that time.

It is probably safe to assume that many of the readers know the symptoms of drowsy driving and that some have been in a near-crash or a crash situation. Most of us have tried to cope with drowsy driving with one of these remedies: turning up the radio, turning on the air conditioning, rolling down the window, singing, or talking to other passengers. The problem is that they help a little, but do not prevent accidents. Pulling the car over for a 10- to 15-minute nap is probably the most effective strategy for dealing with drowsiness while driving. Caffeine does help some with alertness, but is not as good as a nap. Even better, of course, would be sufficient sleep on a regular basis.

The impact of drowsiness on driving performance is multiplied in teenage drivers as they have many strikes against them that increase the likelihood for motor vehicle accidents. Teenage drivers are the least experienced drivers and, therefore, are often poorly equipped to successfully avert car accidents. Their inexperience makes it harder for them to recognize dangerous driving, anticipate hazardous situations, quickly analyze a threat to safety, stay calm, and respond with the correct driving maneuvers to avoid a crash. To make matters worse, teenage drivers and passengers often have less-than-stellar safety habits and are less likely to be wearing a seat belt than more mature drivers. It is also important to recognize that male drivers are twice as likely as female teenage drivers to cause a motor vehicle accident.

Teenagers are used to multitasking and get bored fairly easily when driving a vehicle. Therefore, they often turn to loud music, chatter with their teenage friends and, not infrequently, engage in talking or texting on their cell phones. All of these activities are high-risk behaviors that greatly increase the risk for a car crash.

Teenagers are not supposed to drink alcohol, smoke tobacco or marijuana, or use other illegal substances. Unfortunately, this does not keep them from experimenting. It is not uncommon for teenagers to drive under the influence of one or more mind-altering substances. One can envision quite easily that the addition of sleep deprivation and sleepiness will dramatically increase the risk for a motor vehicle accident.

So what can you do to help teenagers to stay healthy and alive? The first step is to acknowledge that teenage drowsy driving and vehicle crashes are a very serious public health problem. Some risk factors for sleep-related motor vehicle crashes are listed in Table 22-1. You would first want to identify the teenager who is either a driver or frequent passenger in a car with other teenagers. The next step is a simple sleep history that includes total sleep duration, time falling asleep and waking in the morning (school days and weekends), sleep quality, and daytime sleepiness. The use of a standardized questionnaire (ie, Epworth Sleepiness Scale) can be very helpful in getting a sense for the severity of the teenager's sleep deprivation. If the teenager is getting fewer than 7 hours of sleep per night, one would like to know why. Is it hard to fall asleep earlier? What is the bedroom environment like? What types of electronic devices are in the bedroom? These screening questions should be a good starting point for further discussion and exploration of how to improve sleep duration and quality. It is important to engage the teenager actively in problem solving and to avoid a lecturing tone that may be off-putting.

Table 22-1

Features of Adolescents Who Experienced a Motor Vehicle Crash

• Drove more frequently • Drove while sleepy • Drove at night	• Reported poor sleep quality • Used stimulants and tobacco

Adapted from Pizza F, Contardi S, Antognini AB, et al. Sleep quality and motor vehicle crashes in adolescents. *J Clin Sleep Med.* 2010;6(1):41-45.

Suggested Readings

Curry AE, Hafetz J, Kallan MJ, Winston FK, Durbin DR. Prevalence of teen driver errors leading to serious motor vehicle crashes. *Accid Anal Prev.* 2011;43(4):1285-1290.

Klauer SG, Guo F, Simons-Morton BG, et al. Distracted driving and risk of road crashes among novice and experienced drivers. *N Engl J Med.* 2014;370:54-59.

Lucidi F, Devoto A, Bertini M, Braibanti P, Violani C. The effects of sleep debt on vigilance in young drivers: an education/research project in high schools. *J Adolesc.* 2002;25(4):405-414.

Martiniuk AL, Senserrick T, Lo S, et al. Sleep-deprived young drivers and the risk for crash: the DRIVE prospective cohort study. *JAMA Pediatr.* 2013;167(7):647-655.

National Center for Health Statistics. *Data Brief.* No. 37, May 2010. http://www.cdc.gov/nchs/data/databriefs/db37.htm

Pizza F, Contardi S, Antognini AB, et al. Sleep quality and motor vehicle crashes in adolescents. *J Clin Sleep Med.* 2010;6(1):41-45.

SECTION V

NEUROLOGICAL SLEEP DISORDERS

QUESTION 23

What Is Narcolepsy and Do Children Actually Develop This Condition?

Ritu Grewal, MD

Narcolepsy is a rare, chronic disorder characterized by a propensity to fall asleep in situations when an individual would be required to be alert and awake. This is called *hypersomnia* and has many causes.[1] It is commonly encountered in adults, mainly due to inadequate sleep the night before. Children with hypersomnia may be erroneously labeled as lazy or unmotivated. It can have a negative effect on school performance and extracurricular activity. Children may have a hard time waking up in the morning, take excessive daytime naps, and fall asleep in the classroom. Common etiologies of hypersomnia in children are inadequate sleep with poor sleep hygiene; sleep-disordered breathing; circadian rhythm disorders, delayed sleep phase type; psychiatric conditions, such as depression; use of medications and illicit drugs; and narcolepsy.[1]

Narcolepsy is a rare disorder with a prevalence rate of 0.02% to 1.8% in the United States.[2] It is very rarely diagnosed before the age of 5 years. It is present equally in males and females.[3] It typically develops after puberty (between the ages of 15 to 25 years), though many adult patients recall having symptoms before the age of 15 years. About 10% of patients have a first-degree relative with the disorder. It is considered a rapid eye movement (REM) sleep disorder with the intrusion of REM sleep into wakefulness, producing many of the symptoms associated with narcolepsy.

The pathophysiology of narcolepsy involves impaired sleep-wake, and REM/non-REM sleep transitions that appear to be associated with a deficiency of a neurotransmitter, orexin/hypocretin. This neurotransmitter is reduced in many, but not all, patients who have narcolepsy with cataplexy. Orexin promotes wakefulness and suppresses REM sleep. Both genetic and nongenetic factors have been implicated. At the genetic level, HLA subtypes DR2 and DQB1* 0602 have been associated with narcolepsy with cataplexy, with more than 90% of European/White patients testing positive. However, these HLA subtypes have a prevalence of 20% to 35% in the general population, making it difficult to use this as a diagnostic test. An autoimmune mechanism, possible viral infections have been postulated to be responsible in some cases of narcolepsy.[3]

Chidekel AS, ed. *Curbside Consultation in Pediatric Sleep Disorders: 49 Clinical Questions* (pp. 107-110)

Table 23-1

Clinical Features of Narcolepsy

Excessive Daytime Sleepiness
• Initial symptom • Refreshing sleep attacks • Naps involve dreams • Occur during rest or activity
Cataplexy
• Usually occurs after onset of excessive daytime sleepiness • Rapid onset and offset with good memory of the event • Sparing of the diaphragm and ocular muscles
Hypnagogic and Hypnopompic Hallucinations
• Tend to diminish with age • Vivid visual or auditory experiences • Worsened by fatigue and emotion
Sleep Paralysis
• Brief episodes of paralysis at sleep onset or offset • Persistence of REM atonia at wakefulness • Respiratory and ocular muscles are spared • Patient aware of the episode • Distressing

The clinical features of narcolepsy are outlined in Table 23-1. Almost all patients with narcolepsy will have hypersomnia[1] and this is most often the presenting complaint. It may be associated with an irresistible urge to sleep, known as *sleep attacks*. These can occur any time and are usually brief in duration and refreshing for the patient. During these episodes, they may exhibit semi-purposeful or automatic behavior. Other symptoms are cataplexy, sleep paralysis, hypnagogic/hypnopompic hallucinations, and disrupted sleep. Cataplexy is an abrupt loss of muscle tone precipitated by a strong emotion—usually laughter—and is the second most common symptom after hypersomnia. Loss of muscle tone can range from localized sagging of the face, eyelids, or jaw to blurred vision, knee buckling, to complete collapse. During the cataplectic episode, the individual maintains consciousness, and memory is not impaired. It can last from a few seconds to minutes, with complete recovery. It may be confused with atonic seizures, especially in children younger than 5 years. It is rarely the first symptom, but often develops within the first year after the onset of excessive daytime sleepiness. Hypnagogic (sleep onset)/hypnopompic (sleep offset) hallucinations involve vivid auditory or visual hallucinations, often described as dreams. They may be accompanied by sleep paralysis, which is the inability to move or speak for a few seconds at sleep onset or offset. Both of these symptoms can also occur in patients without narcolepsy and represent the intrusion of REM sleep into wakefulness. In addition to these symptoms, nighttime

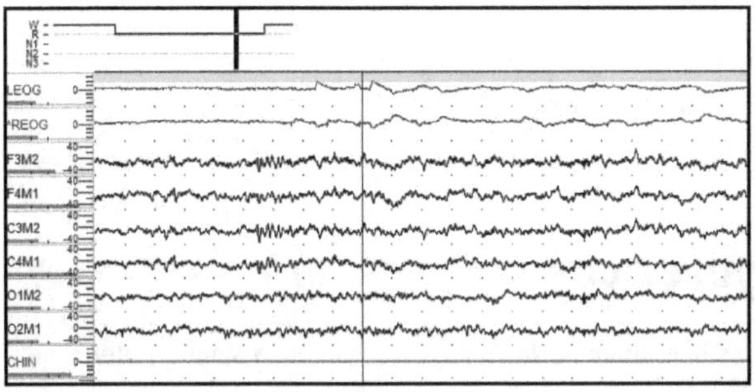

Figure 23-1. Features of REM sleep noted during a multiple sleep latency test in a 15-year-old patient with narcolepsy. The hypnogram at the top of the image shows that the patient entered sleep in stage REM. Sharp eye movements are seen in the electro-oculographic channels along with a low-voltage, mixed-frequency electroenchaphalographic pattern and low amplitude chin electromyography.

sleep is often disrupted with frequent awakenings at night. Narcolepsy may be hard to diagnose in children, as many of the associated symptoms may not be present or easy to elicit.

Children or adolescents with suspected narcolepsy should be referred to a sleep specialist or a pediatric neurologist for diagnosis and management. A complete history should include evaluation of other causes of hypersomnia. In rare cases, narcolepsy can be due to CNS tumors, demyelinating disease, and head trauma. Academic performance, behavioral assessment, and family history should be elicited. Physical examination is usually normal except in cases of secondary narcolepsy. Overnight polysomnogram (PSG), followed by a multiple sleep latency test (MSLT), should be performed in all patients when this disorder is suspected. PSG is useful to rule out sleep-disordered breathing, which is the more common cause of hypersomnia in children.[1] If the PSG is normal, then an MSLT should be done the next day after the patient has slept for at least 6 hours during the PSG, which is a series of 4 scheduled naps for 20 minutes at 2-hour intervals. Diagnostic criteria are mean sleep latency on all 4 naps of less than 8 minutes with 2 sleep onset REM periods (SOREMP). An example of a SOREMP is shown in Figure 23-1. CSF hypocretin levels can be measured if the diagnosis is in doubt, but this is rarely performed in clinical practice.

In one retrospective study, narcolepsy was diagnosed in 51 prepubertal children with a mean age of 7.9 ± 3.1 years.[2] It was present equally in males and females. In 10 children, cataplexy was the presenting symptom. Thirty-eight children had sleep paralysis and 30 had hypnagogic hallucinations. All children had sleep studies; 31 exhibited REM at sleep onset. The mean sleep latency was 1.5 minutes ± 39 seconds on the MSLT. All children had at least 2 SOREMPs. Thirty (65%) families refused any supportive and counseling therapy. Teachers often refused to acknowledge a medical problem. During follow-up, all children presented at least once with depressive symptoms in reaction to their syndrome.

Treatment involves education of the patient, family, and teachers.[2] Behavioral changes include appropriate sleep hygiene with avoidance of sleep deprivation, taking short, refreshing naps, and the avoidance of activities like driving, swimming, or cooking unless the patient is supervised and alert.

Stimulants are used to control the symptoms of excessive daytime sleepiness and REM suppressants to control REM-related phenomena of cataplexy, sleep paralysis, and hallucinations.[4] Stimulant medications like Ritalin (methylphenidate), both short-acting and long-acting, are very well tolerated in the pediatric population. Other medications than can be used are Dexedrine (dextroamphetamine), Adderall (amphetamine), and Provigil (modafinil). Provigil has a lower risk for tolerance and dependence, but is not as efficacious in controlling hypersomnia. It can be combined with Ritalin or Dexedrine. REM suppressants that have been used to control REM-related phenomena, such as cataplexy, are the tricyclic antidepressants and selective serotonin reuptake inhibitors. Xyrem (sodium oxybate) can be used in adolescents. The exact mechanism of action is unknown. It has to be taken twice at night and is very effective in controlling both hypersomnia and REM-related phenomena.

It is important that children with narcolepsy be closely followed as their symptoms may change and doses of medication may need to be adjusted. Narcolepsy should be considered when evaluating children with behavioral and depressive symptoms. Prognosis is very good and most children are able to develop normally and lead productive lives.

References

1. Vendrame M, Havaligi N, Matadeen-Ali C, Adams R, Kothare S. Narcolepsy in children: a single center clinical experience. *Pediatric Neurology.* 2008;38(5):314-320.
2. Guilleminault C, Pelayo R. Narcolepsy in prepubertal children. *Ann Neurol.* 1998;43:135-142.
3. American Academy of Sleep Medicine, ed. Hypersomnias of central origin. In: *The International Classification of Sleep Disorders, Second Edition.* Westchester, IL: American Academy of Sleep Medicine; 2005:79-94.
4. American Academy of Sleep Medicine, ed. Hypersomnias of Central Origin. In: *Case Book of Sleep Medicine.* Westchester, IL: American Academy of Sleep Medicine; 2008:143-155.

24

QUESTION

What Is Restless Legs Syndrome and Do Children Actually Develop This Condition?

Gabor Szuhay, MD

The incidence of restless legs syndrome (RLS) and periodic limb movement disorder (PLMD) in childhood is estimated to be approximately 2%. Therefore, the busy primary pediatrician will likely encounter a couple of children with RLS or PLMD each month. Despite this, most children with RLS will be missed unless the practitioner is aware of the susceptible subpopulations and the subtle signs of its daytime, nighttime, and nocturnal manifestations. PLMD in particular is easily missed, especially if sleep assessment is not a routine part of the child's evaluation.

Briefly, both RLS and PLMD are thought to have a shared pathogenesis. The dopaminergic system originating in the hypothalamus of the A11 pathway to the spinal cord is likely affected. This dopaminergic dysfunction is possibly associated with, or even caused by, the abnormal intracellular iron accumulation in the substantia nigra; this is the only pathological finding on autopsies of patients with RLS to date. Pathological intracellular storage of iron is also suspected based on findings of lower ferritin levels in serum and cerebrospinal fluid of patients with RLS or PLMD, and these lower ferritin levels predict their response to high-dose oral or intravenous iron, as will be discussed later in this chapter.

RLS is one of the most common movement disorders in adults and likely in children as well. It is considered an "involuntary" movement disorder, similar to tics, in which the patient feels an urge to move the limb and suppression of the movement causes escalation of the urge and discomfort; by definition, limb movement at least partially relieves the urge. The diagnosis of RLS relies on subjective patient report; therefore, definite RLS diagnosis can only be established in communicative children. In children, RLS is almost always primary; secondary causes are very rare and will not be discussed here.

Chidekel AS, ed. *Curbside Consultation in Pediatric Sleep Disorders: 49 Clinical Questions* (pp. 111-114)

Symptoms of RLS and PLMD may vary from night to night and week to week, and may relent for months or resolve spontaneously. It is important to note that young children who start experiencing symptoms will often solely complain of leg discomfort and can be misdiagnosed as having growing pains, as the rest of the RLS symptomatology often goes unnoticed unless it is specifically elicited. Additional daytime symptoms include those of sleep disruption. Sleepiness is common and hyperactivity, rebelliousness, and aggression are the cardinal behavioral effects.

For the diagnosis of definite RLS, 4 essential adult criteria must be fulfilled (Table 24-1):

1. The urge to move the limb is often accompanied by a discomfort that the child must be able to describe in his or her own words, such as "spiders crawling," "creepy crawlies," "too much energy," or "electricity." In addition to the legs, arms can be involved also.
2. This urge and discomfort is worse at rest.
3. This urge is worse at night.
4. This urge is relieved at least partially by movement or stretching for as long as the relieving maneuver continues.

If the child cannot describe the discomfort, 2 of the following 3 must be present:

1. A parent or primary relative with RLS
2. Sleep disturbance for age
3. A polysomnography with periodic limb movement index (frequency) above 5 or more movements per hour

Leg discomfort or the urge to move in younger children or infants may manifest as digging their legs into their parents for comfort, asking parents to rub their legs, holding their legs in the air, tucking under their bodies as they are trying to sleep, or putting blankets or stuffed toys on their legs for tension. Importantly, in addition to sleep onset insomnia, children may also have persistence of symptoms into sleep and appear to have sleep maintenance insomnia with tossing and turning, and frequent awakenings.

PLMD implies a periodic movement of the legs—and in addition, though less commonly, the arms—that causes a degree of sleep disruption for age or causes daytime dysfunction (commonly sleepiness or headaches). The periodic limb movement itself is similar to the Babinski response. However, in addition to toe and ankle dorsiflexion, the knees and hips may also flex (triple flexion). The movements are periodic, usually separated by 5 to 90 seconds and occurring in clusters of 3 or more movements with or without arousal (brain activity change) or actual awakening. Children with PLMD have difficulty maintaining sleep, but not exclusively—they may also have sleep onset insomnia, with or without the subjective symptoms of RLS. An increased periodic limb movement index in itself does not necessarily imply PLMD; it may also be a marker for other primary sleep disorders and neurological conditions. Therefore, the primary practitioner will encounter children with increased periodic limb movements in sleep in 2 ways: those with a primary limb movement disorder and those with limb movements secondary to another type of respiratory or nonrespiratory sleep disorder.

Commonly, periodic limb movements are reported as an index: the number of movements per hour of sleep time during the polysomnogram. In children, unlike in adults, a PLMI of 5 or more is considered abnormal. PLMI increases physiologically with age, and PLMI above 10 is found in 30% of adults older than 50 years of age. However, a PLMI of 5 or more is uncommon in children. When one interprets a PLMI that is higher than normal, one should keep in mind that this can be a marker for RLS, but also for other sleep disorders such as narcolepsy or sleep apnea. It is necessary to interview the family about symptoms of RLS or other sleep disorders, as well as family history of PLMD, which is also more common. In sleep-disordered breathing or

Table 24-1

Diagnostic Criteria for Restless Legs Syndrome

Adult Criteria (age 12 and older)
1. Urge to move legs that is often accompanied by uncomfortable and/or unpleasant sensations. 2. These urges and sensations occur during periods of rest or inactivity. 3. Movement such as walking or stretching at least partially relieves these sensations. 4. These sensations either worsen or only occur in the evening or night. 5. There is no better explanation for the condition.
Pediatric Criteria ("1" on its own, or "2" and "3" together, satisfy the criteria)
1. All 4 adult criteria are met *and* the child uses his or her own words to describe leg discomfort. 2. All 4 adult criteria are met *but* the child does not use his or her own words to describe leg discomfort. 3. The child meets at least 2 of the following: a. Sleep disturbance b. Parent or sibling with definite RLS c. Elevated periodic limb movement index (5 or more movements per hour of sleep) on polysomnography

Adapted from American Academy of Sleep Medicine. *International Classification of Sleep Disorders*, 2nd ed. Westchester, IL: American Academy of Sleep Medicine; 2005.

narcolepsy, increased PLMI can be seen and is addressed after the sleep breathing disturbance or narcolepsy are resolved, unless the child meets criteria for RLS, in which case RLS and the coexisting primary sleep disorder can be treated together. A broader differential diagnosis exists as well and is summarized in Table 24-2.

When these disorders are diagnosed, it must be determined whether they are serious enough to warrant treatment, as the symptoms can vary in severity and can fluctuate daily. Measurement of serum ferritin with an iron panel is indicated and, if the ferritin is below 50 ng/mL, supplementation with 3 to 6 mg/kg/day of elemental (free) iron per day is given for a period of 3 months. Favorable response to iron in children can take a few weeks and occur in about 50% to 75% of the cases. Side effects of constipation and abdominal pain may occur. Other medications—such as dopaminergic agents, gabapentin, benzodiazepines, and clonidine—are less commonly used alternatives. Delaying sleep time (maximum symptoms are generally between 9 p.m. to midnight), mild to moderate limb exercise, stretching and, as some patients report, cooling of the spine can also relieve RLS symptoms.

Table 24-2

Differential Diagnosis of Restless Legs Symptoms and Periodic Limb Movements

• Attention deficit hyperactivity disorder • Growing pains • Motor tics	• Musculoskeletal pain • Narcolepsy • Sleep-disordered breathing

Summary

RLS and PLMD are important causes of sleep disruption in children and treatment is effective and relatively safe. Increased PLMI can be a marker of other significant sleep disorders and may influence the expression of many other diseases, clinical course, and outcome. The primary practitioner will need to be vigilant as their manifestations can be subtle, but long-term effects, if left untreated, are akin to other processes with similar sleep disruption.

Suggested Readings

Blum NJ, Mason TBA II. Restless legs syndrome: what is a pediatrician to do? *Pediatrics.* 2007;120(2):438-439.

Hening, WA, Allen RA, Chokroverty S, Early C. *Restless Legs Syndrome.* Philadelphia: Saunders Elsevier; 2009.

Maheswaran M, Kushida CA. Restless legs syndrome in children. *MedGenMed.* 2006;8(2):79. http://www.ncbi.nlm.nih.gov/pmc/articles/PMC1785221/

Picchietti D, et al. Restless legs syndrome: prevalence and impact in children and adolescents—The Peds REST Study. *Pediatrics.* 2007;120(2):253-266.

QUESTION 25

Do Seizures Occur During Sleep and How Commonly Does This Occur?

Gabor Szuhay, MD

The interaction between sleep and epilepsy is well known. Epileptic children frequently experience seizures in drowsiness before sleep, shortly after awakening and—in some epilepsy syndromes—predominantly during sleep. Similarly, sleep deprivation is one of the most frequent causes of breakthrough seizures in children and may be a more common trigger in generalized epilepsy. Prolonged sleep deprivation can elicit seizures in healthy adults without a history of epilepsy. Although such studies in children are not available, a few hours of sleep deprivation the night before can activate epileptiform discharges on the electroencephalogram and aid in diagnosis and classification of seizures in children. There are several ways in which seizures in sleep present to the primary practice. Generally, sleep disruption, restlessness, bedwetting, waking up with confusion or transient neurological dysfunction (rarely Todd's paralysis), morning headaches, feeling sore, lips/tongue bruised in the morning, daytime somnolence, behavioral problems, learning difficulties, or personality changes can be manifestations of nocturnal seizures.

Children with epilepsy also have more sleepiness than nonepileptic children. Even in the absence of sleep disorders, individuals with epilepsy not taking antiepileptic medications (after treatment and a sufficient seizure-free period) had significantly more excessive daytime sleepiness on objective measures. Overall, epileptics had significantly more disrupted sleep, wake periods after sleep onset, decreased deep and rapid eye movement (REM) sleep, and more daytime somnolence—and it was worse in those with uncontrolled seizures. Importantly, sleepiness was more commonly reported in children by their parents than by the children themselves. Obstructive sleep apnea (OSA) is also a possible contributor to sleep disturbance and daytime sleepiness in epileptics. OSA prevalence is higher in children with epilepsy, and limb movements and leg jerks in sleep are also common contributors to sleep disturbance and daytime dysfunction among children with epilepsy as well. In children with epilepsy and even mild OSA, treatment of sleep apnea may significantly improve seizure control. Central apnea is becoming more commonly documented during partial seizures in sleep, and may be an important mechanism in sudden unexplained death in epilepsy.

Chidekel AS, ed. *Curbside Consultation in Pediatric Sleep Disorders: 49 Clinical Questions* (pp. 115-118)

Table 25-1

Epilepsy Syndromes With Prominent Nocturnal Symptomatology

- Benign rolandic epilepsy
- Panayiotopoulos syndrome
- Juvenile myoclonic epilepsy
- Occipital lobe epilepsy
- Nocturnal frontal lobe epilepsy
- Autosomal dominant frontal lobe epilepsy
- Nocturnal temporal lobe epilepsy
- Generalized tonic clonic seizures on awakening
- Infantile spasms
- Lennox-Gastaut syndrome
- Landau-Kleffner syndrome/continuous spike and wave in sleep syndrome

Antiepileptic drugs (AEDs) can also alter the sleep architecture, but this is not a consistent finding with AEDs, although impaired daytime vigilance and sleepiness may be significant side effects. Among the commonly prescribed AEDs, the offenders in order of importance in children are zonisamide, valproic acid, carbamazepine, topiramate, and oxcarbazepine. Levetiracetam and lamotrigine may actually "activate" the child and lamotrigine can cause sleep onset insomnia. Obstructive sleep apnea is not caused by AEDs or epilepsy surgery, but it was observed in 15% of children after vagal nerve stimulator placement for intractable epilepsy.

One must bear in mind that many children, particularly those with intractable epilepsy, are developmentally delayed, and this group of children, even without coexistent epilepsy, are known for having frequent sleep onset and maintenance insomnia; however, many conditions that epileptic children commonly suffer from can also cause sleep disruption or daytime somnolence. Co-sleeping with the worried parent, pain, inability to reposition during obstructive episodes (in cerebral palsy), reflux, anxiety, and depression are common offenders. Tics can occur in all stages of sleep, although complex tics are not common.

Seizures, primarily in sleep (Table 25-1), can be the hallmark of the epilepsy syndrome. However, brain lesions causing symptomatic epilepsies can cause or mimic certain epilepsy syndromes; an EEG will often be distinctive for the particular syndrome, but clinical correlation by a child neurologist should always be obtained. Detailed questioning can help the specialist make a determination regarding whether we are dealing with benign localization related epilepsy—such as benign rolandic epilepsy or Panayiotopoulos syndrome, juvenile myoclonic epilepsy, occipital lobe epilepsy, nocturnal frontal lobe epilepsy and familial autosomal dominant frontal lobe epilepsy, nocturnal temporal lobe epilepsy, generalized tonic clonic seizures on awakening, or if a more malignant epilepsy syndrome is in question, such as one of the epileptic encephalopathies of infancy, Lennox-Gastaut syndrome or Landau-Kleffner syndrome/continuous spike and wave in sleep syndrome. Frequently, and in some cases by definition, developmental regression or plateauing will be present early in malignant epilepsies and should prompt an urgent referral for neurological assessment.

Table 25-2

Common Disorders That Mimic Seizures in Sleep

- Benign sleep myoclonus
- Periodic limb movements of sleep
- Myoclonic jerks
- Bruxism
- Rhythmic sleep movement disorder
- Catathrenia
- Nocturnal dyskinesias
- Alternating leg muscle activation during sleep
- Fragmentary myoclonus
- Paroxysmal nocturnal choking
- Complex parasomnias
- REM sleep behavior disorder

Common disorders that mimic seizures in sleep are listed in Table 25-2. Benign sleep myoclonus, especially of infancy, involves low-amplitude subtle limb twitches that can alternate between limbs, and rarely involve the face, but may last 1 to 2 minutes and be unilateral in rare cases. Periodic limb movements, which can occur in all ages, were discussed in more detail in Question 24. Others include myoclonic jerks at sleep onset (often children report feeling like falling during episodes and may awaken), bruxism (although if the body is not involved, it is unlikely a seizure), rhythmic sleep movement disorder (commonly 2 to 3 Hz head banging and body rocking that lessens or stops with gentle tactile stimulation), catathrenia (sleep moaning on exhalation, can also stop with tactile stimulation) and, less commonly, nocturnal dyskinesias (difficult to distinguish from seizures; video electroenphalography (EEG) monitoring may be necessary). Less common sleep movements, such as alternating leg muscle activation during sleep and fragmentary myoclonus, are even less common in children. Nocturnal paroxysmal choking is also exceedingly rarely reported in children. Parasomnias (night terrors and sleepwalking, hybrid spells, or confusional arousals, more so than nightmares) are very common and sometimes difficult to distinguish from seizures, especially frontal lobe seizures. Finally, children who are dreaming may have rapid eye movements that the inexperienced parent may mistake for epilepsy; some children may have an unusually active REM sleep with hypnic jerks of the limbs. REM behavioral disorder can be associated with complex behaviors, is often aggressive in nature, is extremely rare in children, and is commonly associated with narcolepsy.

Summary

Seizures, whether genetic or caused by a brain lesion, can have similar presentation and may mimic more benign nocturnal phenomena. A sleep-deprived EEG is essential as the first diagnostic test with provoking maneuvers (photic stimulation, hyperventilation) until the child is evaluated by a sleep specialist or neurologist; often, overnight or multiple night monitoring is necessary. If seizures are strongly suspected, a video EEG is a better choice over polysomnography. Sleep is disrupted in children with an epileptogenic brain, especially with uncontrolled seizures, and may involve sleep breathing disorders or sleep movement disorders, and may indirectly worsen seizure frequency and daytime function. The approach should be comprehensive and all offending disorders should be addressed to optimize developmental outcome.

Suggested Readings

Al-Biltagi MA. Childhood epilepsy and sleep. *World J Clin Pediatr.* 2014;3(3):45-53.

Eriksson SH. Epilepsy and sleep. *Current Opinion in Neurology.* 2011;24(2):171-176.

Kotagal P, Yardi N. The relationship between sleep and epilepsy. *Semin Pediatr Neurol.* 2008;15(2):42-49.

Kothare, SV, Kotagal, S. *Sleep in Childhood Neurological Disorders.* New York: Demos Medical Publishing; 2011.

Pellock, J; Dodson, WE; Bourgeois, BFD. *Pediatric Epilepsy: Diagnosis and Therapy, 3rd Edition.* New York: Demos Medical Publishing; 2008.

QUESTION 26

What Are Some of the Other More Common Neurological Problems That Can Influence Sleep?

Gabor Szuhay, MD

Sleep disorders generally have been better characterized in the pediatric population in decades, but the nature of sleep problems in pediatric subpopulations, such as pediatric neurological patients, is still largely understudied. In general, the major risk factors for sleep problems in neurologically impaired children are independent of their neurological conditions and are more important in causing sleep problems than those associated with their underlying neurological disorder. The spectrum of sleep problems range from insomnia and sleep-wake cycle disturbance to sleep-disordered breathing and narcolepsy. Some subpopulations in pediatric neurology may have more pronounced or multiple risk factors, but often the children's sleep problems are initially ascribed to their underlying condition or treatment effect. Chronic pulmonary disease, reflux, pain, and psychological disorders are very common in this population. We will briefly discuss major sleep disorders and ways that neurologically impaired children can be affected.

Among the sleep cycle disorders, delayed sleep phase syndrome is very common in teenagers—it can restrict sleep time and cause daytime sleepiness, and it can exacerbate existing neurological conditions, such as epilepsy, headaches, behavioral problems, or learning disabilities. After concussions, sleep-wake cycle disorder is common, as is insomnia—likely due to autonomic nervous system damage. It is usually transient for a few months and responds to behavioral therapy and melatonin. Behavioral therapy of the patient and the family may be sufficient, but melatonin can be useful, too, until a more permanent solution is in place.

Insomnia, whether sleep onset or maintenance, is common in the pediatric neurological population. It can be primary or secondary to other sleep disorders. Insomnia is often multifactorial in the cognitively challenged population and is often a result of comorbid psychological conditions in intellectually normal and slightly below-average children. Intellectually challenged children may not recognize the need to conform to sleep-wake cycles and the abnormal brain function may also prevent cueing an appropriate sleep schedule. This is particularly impaired in some blind children, who have a free-running circadian rhythm; without natural light cueing the 24-hour sleep-wake

Chidekel AS, ed. *Curbside Consultation in Pediatric Sleep Disorders: 49 Clinical Questions* (pp. 119-121)

cycle, they may require melatonin, but can also respond to behavioral therapy in selected cases. In autism, whether high- or low-functioning, insomnia is almost the norm. As in nonautistic delayed children, behavioral therapies may be sufficient, but melatonin or other therapeutics may be necessary. In children with anxiety disorders or depression, cognitive behavioral therapy is effective and should always be favored over medications.

With the exception of some specific subpopulations of neurologically impaired children, adenotonsillar hypertrophy and snoring remain the major predictors for sleep-disordered breathing. Obesity, especially common in some patients with neuromuscular disease, is also an important risk factor. For this reason, sleep-disordered breathing and, specifically, obstructive apnea is more common in the ages from 2 to 8, when tonsillar size peaks. However, multiple risk factors can culminate to render children highly susceptible for sleep apnea at any age (eg, Down syndrome, obesity, craniofacial features, adenotonsillar hypertrophy, and hypotonia). More specifically, upper airway hypotonia can culminate into multilevel upper airway obstruction, sometimes necessitating tracheostomy to achieve upper airway patency in sleep. Other neurological diseases may have more common single-risk factors. In mucopolysaccharidosis, tonsils are frequently enlarged and some children with myelomeningocele have sleep apnea even without neuroradiological evidence of posterior fossa compromise or Chiari II malformation. In cerebral palsy—especially quadriplegic cerebral palsy—in addition to other risk factors, children may not be able to reposition themselves to relieve episodic upper airway compromise. In neuromuscular disorders, more commonly and predictably in congenital muscle disease—specifically in Duchenne muscular dystrophy and in spinal muscular atrophy—sleep apnea can be predicted with some certainty with advancing weakness. In other conditions, such as myasthenia gravis outside of exacerbations, sleep apnea is still more common in obese patients. Sleep disruption in itself can cause daytime behaviors of hyperactivity, aggression, and rebelliousness. Sleep has been extensively studied in attention deficit hyperactivity disorder, and findings show that daytime sleepiness and the previously mentioned daytime behaviors are not particularly predictive of sleep-disordered breathing; however, as is discussed in Question 24 in more detail, RLS and PLMD are more commonly the cause of sleep disruption. Pediatric headache patients have nonspecific sleep disturbances, mostly from the same behavioral problems that predispose them to headaches; however, sleep apnea in thin, young males with idiopathic intracranial hypertension (pseudotumor cerebri) is more common than would be predicted, but obesity is still the most important predictor of sleep apnea in patients with intracranial hypertension. Children with structural lesions of the brainstem, including tumors or such metabolic disorders as mitochondrial diseases or demyelination in multiple sclerosis during exacerbations, can develop sleep apnea, but apnea is rarely the only neurological symptom of the disease. Adenotonsillectomy, when indicated, adequately treats sleep-disordered breathing in the vast majority of nonobese children, and this may be true even in some of the most impaired (eg, in children with quadriplegic cerebral palsy). In some syndromes or in children with severe hypotonia or weakness, this may not be as effective, however. Even neurologically impaired children can respond to desensitization for continuous positive airway pressure, as can their normal counterparts, but, in some populations, this may not prove to be feasible even after desensitization. Also, in neurological conditions that are difficult to control, in which even milder forms of sleep-disordered breathing are suspected to play a role, clinicians may choose to treat the disease.

Daytime somnolence is common among handicapped children, but should be qualified and quantified the same way as in their normal counterparts. For example, in myotonic dystrophy, children may appear somnolent, but this may not be supported by MSLT studies. In children with seizures, daytime somnolence can be multifactorial, due to frequent sleep disruption from seizures and interictal discharges, but the epileptogenic brain may itself be predisposing to daytime somnolence (see Question 25). Narcolepsy, whether associated with cataplexy or more commonly not, is more common than recognized, and more common than all nonstatic white matter disorders combined. Some neurological syndromes may be specifically associated with narcolepsy, such as Norrie disease, Coffin-Lowry syndrome, and Prader-Willi syndrome. Narcolepsy can be initiated by minor head trauma, as well as by sleep apnea, stress, or drug abuse. It can be secondary to almost any condition that affects the hypothalamus, from infection to ADEM, and from tumors to radiation and even hydrocephalus. Perhaps more so than with other symptoms, daytime somnolence and sleep disruption are almost always ascribed to the underlying neurological condition. The workup for narcolepsy is discussed elsewhere, but secondary forms can be difficult to diagnose and some children may not meet strict criteria on first attempt. Other syndromes of hypersomnolence—for example, the rare Kleine-Levin syndrome—are difficult to diagnose in mentally handicapped children; cyclical bizarre behavior may be the only clue for derealization, and hypersexuality is rare in younger or handicapped children. Other cyclical neurobehavioral disorders may also mimic Kleine-Levin syndrome, such as Sydenham's chorea, Pediatric Autoimmune Neuropsychiatric Disorders Associated with Streptococcal Infections, or pediatric bipolar or thought disorder; the latter are also difficult to recognize in handicapped children. Treatment of daytime somnolence in children is similar to treatment of their normal counterparts; however, stimulants should be used carefully in certain subgroups, such as epileptics and children with tics—Modafinil is safer.

Among sleep movement disorders, RLS and PLMD have been more recently recognized as frequent in attention deficit hyperactivity disorder (see Question 24). Other sleep movement disorders, such as rhythmic sleep movement disorder—characterized by 2 to 3 Hz body rocking, head banging, or more complex repetitive behaviors—are common in the delayed population and in autism. Tics can occur in all stages of sleep, although complex tics are almost never seen. Rhythmic sleep movement disorders are benign, bed padding can prevent banging, and transient use of melatonin can be effective if the condition is disruptive.

Parasomnias are understudied in children, but are common among the developmentally delayed population and in all children who have sleep disruption, regardless of cause. Frontal lobe epilepsy and its less severe subtypes can mimic parasomnias or trigger them; these and other seizure types in sleep were discussed in Question 25.

Summary

Sleep disorders affect neurologically impaired children more commonly and some more severely; some neurological disorders display unique sleep disorders that the clinician must be aware of. Sleep disorders may alter the presentation, course, and outcome of neurological disorders and, in themselves, may have long-term morbidities. Treatment of sleep problems in neurologically impaired children can be challenging, but, in general, the treating clinicians follow similar diagnostic and treatment approaches as in normal children.

Suggested Readings

Dorris L, Scott N, Zuberi S, Gibson N, Espie C. Sleep problems in children with neurological disorders. *Dev Neurorehabil.* 2008;11(2):95-114.

Galland BC, Elder DE, Taylor B. Interventions with a sleep outcome for children with cerebral palsy and post-traumatic brain injury: a systematic review. *Sleep Med Rev.* 2012;16(6):561-573.

Ming X, Walters AS: Autism spectrum disorders, attention deficit/hyperactivity disorder, and sleep disorders. *Curr Opin in Pulm Med.* 2009;15(6):578-584.

Malow BA, Byars K, Johnson K, et al. A Practice Pathway for the Identification, Evaluation and Management of Insomnia in Children and Adolescents With Autism Spectrum Disorders. *Pediatrics*;130:S106-S124.

SECTION VI

PEDIATRIC OBSTRUCTIVE SLEEP APNEA SYNDROME

QUESTION 27

What Is Obstructive Sleep Apnea Syndrome?

Lynn A. D'Andrea, MD and Louella Amos, MD

Definition and Epidemiology

Obstructive sleep apnea syndrome (OSAS) is a sleep-related breathing disorder characterized by partial or complete upper airway obstruction, which can be intermittent and/or prolonged, and which "disrupts normal ventilation during sleep, normal sleep patterns, or both."[1] In general, 1% to 5% of children have OSAS.[2] Often, these children have adenotonsillar hypertrophy (Figure 27-1). Adenoid tissue grows most rapidly between infancy and early childhood, with regression after age 6 years. Tonsils are largest from age 4 to 10 years and start to atrophy with the onset of puberty. Obesity (BMI > 95th percentile) is another comorbidity associated with OSAS. Other risk factors for pediatric OSAS are listed in Table 27-1.

Pathophysiology

Airflow limitation occurs because of fixed obstruction (eg, adenotonsillar hypertrophy), dynamic airway closure (eg, decreased pharyngeal tone), or a combination of the two. The airway collapse in OSAS is similar to what happens when you try to drink a thick milkshake through a flimsy straw. Pharyngeal tone decreases during sleep, particularly during rapid eye movement (REM) sleep when there is global muscle atonia. In overweight children, increased adipose tissue in the pharyngeal structures and subcutaneous tissues in the neck result in intrinsic narrowing and extrinsic compression, respectively, of the airway lumen.

Chidekel AS, ed. *Curbside Consultation in Pediatric Sleep Disorders: 49 Clinical Questions* (pp. 125-128)

Figure 27-1. The black arrow identifies the enlarged adenoid pad resulting in nasopharyngeal narrowing.

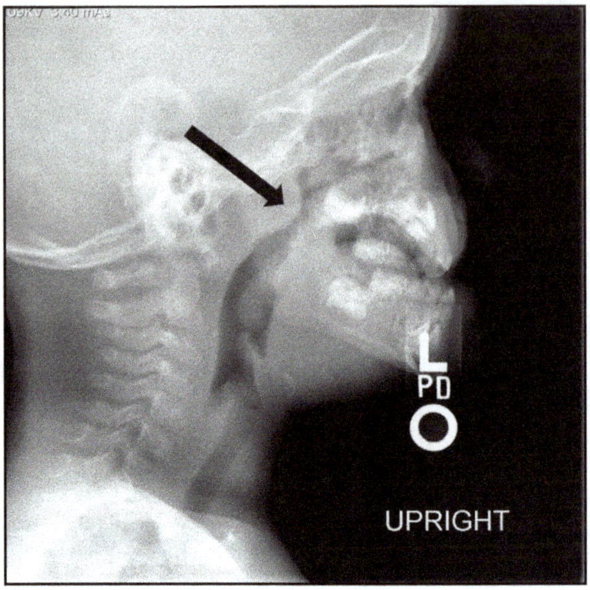

Table 27-1

Pediatric Obstructive Sleep Apnea Syndrome Risk Factors

- Adenotonsillar hypertrophy
- Obesity
- Craniofacial abnormalities and associated syndromes (eg, Down syndrome, Pierre Robin sequence)
- Abnormal neuromuscular tone
    - Muscular dystrophy
    - Static encephalopathy
- Black background
- Male gender
- History of prematurity
- Family history of OSAS

Clinical Presentation and Diagnosis

Parents usually report that their child has audible snoring and "stops breathing" (ie, obstructive apneas). Because of the sleep disruption caused by OSAS, children may have worsening sleep terrors, excessive daytime sleepiness, and/or daytime behavior problems with hyperactivity. Nighttime bedwetting has been associated with OSAS, although no clear causation has been proven. These and other signs and symptoms of OSAS are listed in Table 27-2.

Table 27-2

Pediatric Obstructive Sleep Apnea Syndrome Signs and Symptoms

- Loud snoring
- Witnessed apneas/gasping
- Mouth breathing
- Labored breathing with paradoxic respiratory efforts
- Diaphoresis
- Morning headaches
- Restless sleep
- Morning tiredness and daytime sleepiness
- Daytime hyperactivity
- Behavioral problems
- Parasomnias (sleep terrors, enuresis)

Clinical history alone, obtained by parent-driven questionnaires or a clinician, poorly predicts the diagnosis of OSAS; therefore, objective testing is necessary. Polysomnography is the gold standard for diagnosing OSAS. This and other forms of objective testing will be discussed in Questions 29 and 47.

Why Treat Obstructive Sleep Apnea Syndrome?

Consolidated sleep is essential for cognitive development, growth, and cardiovascular health. The sleep fragmentation and intermittent hypoxia caused by OSAS has deleterious consequences on neurocognitive function. After treatment of OSAS, school performance, attention capacity, behavior, and quality of life improve. OSAS also impairs somatic growth, as evidenced by an increase in growth parameters and biomarkers, such as insulin-like growth factor-I, after treatment of OSAS with adenotonsillectomy.[3] Hypertension and autonomic dysregulation during wakefulness and sleep are the reported cardiovascular sequelae of untreated OSAS.[4] These effects may be due to the sympathetic surges and inflammatory response cascade in the vascular endothelium associated with chronic nocturnal obstructive respiratory events. Improvement in cognition and growth biomarkers can be seen within months of OSAS treatment.[3,5]

Surgical Treatment

Children older than 1 year of age with OSAS and adenotonsillar hypertrophy most commonly undergo adenotonsillectomy, which is often curative or, at the very least, decreases the severity of the disease. Obesity, male gender, severe preoperative OSAS, and craniofacial abnormalities increase the risk for residual OSAS after surgery. The most frequently reported postoperative complications include pain, nausea, vomiting, dehydration, and bleeding. Adenoid regrowth is more likely in those who have their adenoids removed before reaching 6 years of age.

Partial tonsillectomy is a technique that reduces the postoperative morbidity associated with traditional tonsillectomy. Partial tonsillectomy results in less pain, decreased occurrence of bleeding, and earlier recovery; however, there is also increased risk of tonsillar regrowth.

Other more complex airway surgeries employed by pediatric otolaryngologists to optimize airway patency include nasal turbinate reduction, lingual tonsillectomy, palatopharyngoplasty, hyoid suspension, and genioglossal advancement.

Medical Treatment

Depending on the etiology, certain nonsurgical interventions may also be helpful. In overweight children, weight loss may help not only their sleep-disordered breathing, but also their overall health. Topical nasal steroids and leukotriene inhibitors have been shown to shrink adenoid tissue and treat mild OSAS. Rapid maxillary expansion is an orthodontic procedure that treats maxillary constriction and dental malocclusion by opening the midpalatal suture, thereby widening the narrow hard palate.

Continuous positive airway pressure (CPAP) stents open the upper airway by delivering positive pressure into the airway through a mask. This is an option for children who are not surgical candidates, who have residual OSAS after surgery, or whose parents choose the nonsurgical approach. CPAP effectively treats OSAS, but there are limitations. Because of the constantly changing facial structure of young children, maintaining an appropriate mask fit can be difficult. Adherence to therapy is another issue, particularly in young children who may not tolerate the setup or adolescents who may not feel they need nightly treatment. Complications of CPAP use are usually secondary to an inappropriate mask fit and include skin breakdown on the face and maxillary retrusion. Close monitoring by the sleep specialist is required to avoid these complications.

Summary

Pediatric OSAS is common enough that a health care provider should know how to recognize the signs and symptoms, which would warrant further evaluation, objective testing, and subsequent treatment. This is important because of the neurocognitive consequences, impaired mood, altered somatic growth, and cardiovascular abnormalities observed in children with OSAS.

References

1. American Academy of Sleep Medicine. *International Classification of Sleep Disorders, 2nd Edition: Diagnostic and Coding Manual.* Westchester, IL: American Academy of Sleep Medicine, 2005.
2. Marcus CL, Brooks LJ, Ward SD, et al. Technical report, diagnosis and management of childhood obstructive sleep apnea syndrome. *Pediatrics.* 2012;130:e714-e755.
3. Selimoglu E, Selimoglu MA, Orbak Z. Does adenotonsillectomy improve growth in children with obstructive adenotonsillar hypertrophy? *J Int Medical Res.* 2003;31:84-87.
4. O'Brien LM, Gozal D. Autonomic dysfunction in children with sleep-disordered breathing. *Sleep* 2005;28:747-752.
5. Friedman BC, Hendeles-Amitai A, Kozminsky E, et al. Adenotonsillectomy improves neurocognitive function in children with obstructive sleep apnea syndrome. *Sleep.* 2003;26:999-1005.

QUESTION 28

Which Children Are at Increased Risk for Pediatric Obstructive Sleep Apnea Syndrome?

Suzanne E. Beck, MD

Snoring and obstructive sleep apnea syndrome (OSAS) are common in children and can occur at any age. In general, there are 3 clinically distinct populations of children at increased risk for OSAS:

1. Preschool and school-aged children who snore, have adenotonsillar hypertrophy, and may or may not have behavioral problems such as hyperactivity or inattention/poor school performance.
2. Older school-aged children and adolescents who snore, may be overweight, and have excessive daytime sleepiness, school problems, or behavioral problems.
3. Special populations with comorbid medical conditions, such as Down syndrome, neuromuscular disorders, or craniofacial anomalies like cleft palate or retrognathia, or which are from high-risk groups. During routine pediatric care, all children should be screened for snoring and further evaluated if OSAS is suspected (Table 28-1).

Children Who Snore Are at Increased Risk of Obstructive Sleep Apnea

Snoring is the hallmark symptom of obstructive sleep apnea syndrome (OSAS) in children and is very common. Almost all children who have OSAS snore; however, not all children who snore have OSAS. The prevalence of habitual snoring is 12% to 15% among preschool and school-aged children, whereas the prevalence of OSAS in the general pediatric population in most studies is

Chidekel AS, ed. *Curbside Consultation in Pediatric Sleep Disorders: 49 Clinical Questions* (pp. 129-134)

Table 28-1

Which Children Are at Risk for Obstructive Sleep Apnea?

- Toddlers/children who snore, have adenotonsillar hypertrophy, and have daytime symptoms, such as inattention, hyperactivity, poor school performance
- Children/adolescents who snore, may be overweight/obese, and have daytime symptoms, such as poor school performance and daytime sleepiness
- Special populations of children with craniofacial anomalies (eg, cleft palate, retrognathia, achondroplasia), comorbid medical conditions (eg, Down syndrome, Prader-Willi syndrome, neuromuscular disorders), or who are at high risk due to low socioeconomic status, prematurity, or race

only 0.8% to 2.8%. Therefore, only a fraction of those who snore actually have OSAS. The clinician should consider further evaluation in children who snore and have other risk factors for OSAS as outlined in the recent American Academy of Pediatrics (AAP) clinical practice guideline on the diagnosis and management of pediatric obstructive sleep apnea. Because OSAS is common, and if left untreated could have severe complications, all children and adolescents should be screened for snoring and OSAS as part of their routine health care visit. When snoring or other signs, symptoms, or risk factors for OSAS are present, further evaluation is indicated.

It is worth noting that snoring can be underreported in children, and some studies have shown that OSAS is probably underdiagnosed in children. It is important to keep in mind that whether a child's snoring is reported at a routine health care visit is dependent on the perception of the caregiver and the vigilance of the clinician. Snoring may not be reported because it may not be heard or perceived as abnormal. Snoring may be quiet or absent in infants or in children with neuromuscular disorders. Therefore, the clinician should ask open-ended questions about breathing problems during sleep. When screening patients for snoring or sleep disordered breathing, I tend to open with, "How is your child's breathing during sleep?" or "Is there anything that worries you about your child's breathing while sleeping?" I follow up with, "Is the breathing quiet or do you hear any sounds?", "Is the breathing labored or the sleep restless?", "Does your child sleep in unusual positions?", and "Is there any snoring?" If the answer to "Is there any snoring?" is negative, I ask, "Can you hear your child breathe or make any noises at all while sleeping?"

Other nighttime symptoms associated with OSAS are labored breathing, gasping, snorting, observed episodes of apnea, sleeping in a seated position or with the neck hyperextended, and secondary enuresis.

OSAS is defined by what happens during sleep—a disorder of breathing during sleep characterized by prolonged partial upper airway obstruction and/or intermittent complete obstruction (obstructive apnea) that disrupts normal ventilation during sleep and normal sleep patterns—as defined by the American Thoracic Society; however, there may be daytime symptoms associated with OSAS. Daytime symptoms are nonspecific and include hyperactivity, behavioral problems, emotional lability, inattention, poor school performance, excessive daytime sleepiness, failure to thrive/poor weight gain, morning headache, noisy breathing, and mouth breathing. Hyperactivity is the most common daytime symptom reported in children with OSAS, and children with OSAS have a 3-fold higher increase in behavior and neurocognitive symptoms compared to controls. OSAS is more common in children with symptoms of mild attention deficit hyperactivity disorder (ADHD) compared to children with significant ADHD or controls without ADHD, highlighting that children with OSAS may be mislabeled or misdiagnosed with ADHD. In my experience as a clinician, most parents report that overtired children tend to be more hyperactive or act out, rather than act "sleepy," and usually do not request to take a nap. It is, therefore, important to consider evaluation for OSAS in children with mild ADHD-like symptoms.

Excessive daytime sleepiness is the most common reported daytime symptom in adults with OSAS; however, it is uncommonly reported in prepubertal children with OSAS. When carefully questioned and evaluated, some children with OSAS are sleepier than children without OSAS. Excessive sleepiness is more common in overweight children with and without OSAS and more common in older or obese children with OSAS than in younger children with OSAS. Noisy breathing and mouth breathing are usually the result of adenoidal hypertrophy in the preschool-aged child. Morning headaches are uncommon in children with OSAS, but are a common manifestation of sleep-disordered breathing in children with neuromuscular disorders, likely related to carbon dioxide retention, and require further evaluation when present. The clinician should be astute in recognizing daytime behaviors and symptoms in children that could be linked to problems during sleep.

Physical Exam Findings in Children With Obstructive Sleep Apnea Syndrome Are Nonspecific

Adenotonsillar hypertrophy is associated with OSAS and removal can be curative in most otherwise healthy children. The size of tonsils on physical examination does not predict the presence or severity of OSAS, but size as measured more precisely in research studies does correlate with OSAS. It is believed that anatomic factors are a primary (but not the sole) cause of OSAS in young children who snore and adenotonsillectomy is the recommended first-line treatment. OSAS can persist in a minority of patients after adenotonsillectomy, indicating that clinical follow up is important. Other physical exam findings are usually normal or nonspecific. Children with the following conditions deserve special attention when it comes to assessing risk for OSAS, as each are at increased risk of OSAS:

- Obesity or failure to thrive
- Hypertension
- High-arched palate
- Adenoidal facies
- Craniofacial anomalies, such as cleft palate
- Retrognathia
- Children with neuromuscular weakness or syndromes, such as Down syndrome, muscular dystrophy, achondroplasia, or spina bifida

Children Who Are Obese Have a Higher Risk of Having Obstructive Sleep Apnea Syndrome

In a recent study, childhood obesity was a strong independent risk factor for having mild or moderate OSAS. Obese children with OSAS are more likely to manifest excessive daytime sleepiness and have increased inflammatory markers, similar to adults, indicating that metabolic factors may play a role in the pathogenesis of OSAS similar to that in adults. Adenotonsillectomy is still considered first-line therapy for obese children with OSAS and adenotonsillar hypertrophy, as the obstructive apnea-hypopnea index may improve significantly following surgery. It is important to note that OSAS may persist in obese children after adenotonsillectomy and would require further treatment, such as continuous positive airway pressure (CPAP) during sleep; therefore, clinical follow up and polysomnography are important in this population.

Children With Comorbid Medical Conditions and Syndromes Involving Alteration in Craniofacial Structure or Muscle Tone Are at Increased Risk of Obstructive Sleep Apnea

It is beyond the scope of this chapter to discuss, or even list, every syndrome or anatomic abnormality associated with a higher risk of OSAS in children. It is important to recognize treatable causes of behavioral, cognitive, and developmental impairment in children with underlying syndromes associated with neurocognitive impairment or craniofacial anomalies. Treatable causes, such as obstructive sleep apnea, may go overlooked, contributing significantly to the morbidity often associated solely to the underlying syndrome.

Children With Down Syndrome Are at Increased Risk of Obstructive Sleep Apnea

These children are at increased risk because of innate features of the syndrome, such as glossoptosis, maxillary hypoplasia, and hypotonia. The prevalence of OSAS in children with Down syndrome is very high and is often present in children in whom it was not suspected. Hypotonia associated with Down syndrome (as well as with other disorders) can cause profound physiological aberrations associated with obstructive events, such as a higher degree of upper airway collapsibility and increased thoracoabdominal asynchrony, causing lower functional residual capacity and resultant hypoxemia compared to typical children. Children with Down syndrome are more likely to have comorbid conditions that place them at higher risk for OSAS, such as higher incidences of being overweight or obese, having a lingual tonsil, and having hypothyroidism. Children with Down syndrome are more likely to have brain stem abnormalities associated with autonomic dysregulation, accounting for some of the increased prevalence of OSAS. Untreated OSAS may be a contributor to the pulmonary hypertension noted in Down syndrome. The AAP has recognized the importance of OSAS in Down syndrome and has included screening for OSAS in their policy on Health Supervision for Children With Down Syndrome. Because many of the behavioral and neurocognitive sequelae of untreated OSAS overlap with the developmental deficits associated with Down syndrome (and other syndromes), it is important for the clinician to identify treatable causes that may improve overall health and development of the child.

Children With Prader-Willi Syndrome

These children are also at higher risk of having OSAS because of hypotonia in infancy, obesity, and ventilatory control abnormalities as the child grows. In addition, treatment with growth hormone may accelerate lymphoid hyperplasia. It is our practice to screen all infants and children with Prader-Willi syndrome for OSAS before and during treatment with growth hormone. It is our practice to treat (even very mild) OSAS appropriately by adenotonsillectomy or CPAP before initiating or continuing growth hormone therapy and to follow these children regularly.

Children With Hypotonia or Neuromuscular Disorders Are Vulnerable to Obstructive Sleep Apnea Syndrome

Sleep-disordered breathing often precedes diurnal respiratory failure in this population. Children with neuromuscular disease are at risk for both alveolar hypoventilation (due to breathing at low lung volumes and the development of atelectasis and mucus plugging), as well as upper airway obstruction. There seems to be a bimodal presentation of sleep-disordered breathing in patients with Duchenne muscular dystrophy (DMD), with OSAS found in the first decade and hypoventilation more commonly seen in the second decade. Snoring may be light or not present. The child may complain of fatigue due to increasing numbers of nocturnal awakenings, daytime sleepiness, morning headache, and sometimes vomiting. Current guidelines of the care of a patient with DMD recommend an annual evaluation for sleep-disordered breathing be performed in these patients, starting from the time they are wheelchair users and/or when clinically indicated, and that a review of sleep quality and symptoms of sleep disordered breathing be performed at every patient encounter. The guidelines also suggest the use of nighttime ventilatory support when daytime $PCO_2 > 50$ mm Hg and $SpO_2 < 92\%$. It is important for the front-line clinician to recognize that OSAS and sleep-disordered breathing may be present in asymptomatic infants and children with neuromuscular disorders and have a low threshold to encourage further evaluation and appropriate treatment because this may improve the child's quality of life.

Infants and Children With Myelomeningocele

Those affected with this common serious birth defect, often associated with an Arnold-Chiari malformation of the brainstem, are at increased risk of sleep-disordered breathing, which, in this population, can be due central apnea, obstructive apnea, central hypoventilation, sleep-exacerbated restrictive lung disease, or a mixture of these. Each requires different specific treatment. The symptoms of untreated sleep-disordered breathing, such as cognitive and developmental impairment, may overlap with symptoms associated with spina bifida itself. In addition, because of the frequency of doctor visits, children with spina bifida (as well as other children with complex medical care and routines) may avoid what seems like unnecessary evaluation. The clinician should be vigilant in screening for signs and symptoms of OSAS in this vulnerable population and advocate for further evaluation when indicated.

Infants and Children With Craniofacial Syndromes or Syndromes Associated With Craniofacial Anomalies

These patients are at a higher risk for OSAS. There are numerous syndromes, including Pierre Robin sequence, Treacher Collins syndrome, Goldenhar syndrome, and achondroplasia, to name a few, that are associated with craniofacial anomalies placing the infant or child at risk for OSAS. Infants and children with cleft palate or any syndrome associated with retrognathia, micrognathia, midface hypoplasia, maxillary insufficiency, or high-arched palate should be screened for OSAS. Importantly, children with a cleft palate or children with underlying low muscle tone may not snore. Numerous specialists follow many of these children and not all may be aware of the risk for OSAS. The pediatrician should advocate for evaluation by a sleep specialist to diagnose and treat OSAS to improve overall developmental and neurocognitive outcomes in this population.

The prevalence of OSAS is higher in children with sickle cell disease (SCD) as compared with the general pediatric population. Factors related to SCD that are thought to be important include the excessive lymphoid hyperplasia associated with SCD, as well as socioeconomic factors. In addition, the Black race, in itself, may be a risk factor for OSAS. Untreated OSAS may have significant sequelae in children with SCD due to the effects of hypoxemia, hypercarbia, and respiratory acidosis on polymerization of Hemoglobin S and subsequent vaso-occlusive crisis and morbidity. Therefore, OSAS should be recognized and treated in these vulnerable children.

Other At-Risk Groups

Infants and children who are from lower socioeconomic backgrounds, were born prematurely, or are of Black descent are at a higher risk for OSAS. The front-line clinician should keep these factors in mind when screening for OSAS.

Suggested Readings

Bull M. Committee on Genetics. Health supervision for children with Down syndrome. *Pediatrics*. 2011;128(2):393-406. doi:10.1542/peds.2011-1605.

Finder JD, Birnkrant D, Carl J, et al. Respiratory care of the patient with Duchenne muscular dystrophy: ATS consensus statement. *Am J Crit Care Med.* 2004:17(4):456-465.

Kirk VG, Morielli A, Gozal, G, Marcus, et al. Treatment of sleep-disordered breathing in children with myelomeningocele. *Pediatr Pulmonol.* 2000;30:445-452.

Marcus CL, Brooks LJ, Draper KA, et al. Clinical practice guidelines. Diagnosis and management of childhood obstructive sleep apnea syndrome. *Pediatrics.* 2012;130:1-9.

Marcus CL, Brooks LJ, Ward SD, et al. Technical report. Diagnosis and management of childhood obstructive sleep apnea syndrome. *Pediatrics.* 2012;130:1-42.

Section on Pediatric Pulmonology, Subcommittee on Obstructive Sleep Apnea Syndrome. American Academy of Pediatrics. Clinical practice guideline diagnosis and management of childhood obstructive sleep apnea syndrome. *Pediatrics.* 2002;109(4):704-712.

QUESTION 29

How Is Pediatric Obstructive Sleep Apnea Syndrome Diagnosed?

Louella Amos, MD and Lynn A. D'Andrea, MD

Diagnosing pediatric obstructive sleep apnea syndrome (OSAS) entails a detailed clinical history, comprehensive physical exam, and diagnostic tools. The clinical evaluation alone, however, is insufficient and often inaccurate in predicting who does and does not have OSAS. Objective diagnostics, usually in the form of polysomnography, are necessary to accurately diagnose this sleep disorder.

Parents or siblings provide most of the sleep history. Snoring is the most commonly reported symptom and can be loud and continuous or intermittent. We ask parents if they can hear their children snore through a closed door to help define the loudness or severity of the snoring. Mouth breathing may be present, especially if the child has chronic nasal congestion. Family members may report respiratory pauses followed by gasping or choking during sleep. Sometimes, we mimic an obstructive apnea episode for the parents and ask them if that is what they hear at night; respiratory pauses during sleep can be normal, so it is important to distinguish a normal pause from a pathologic obstructive pause. Parents may bring video- or audio-recordings of their child sleeping to show the clinician what they observe at night. Other associated signs and symptoms include diaphoresis, enuresis, morning headaches, daytime sleepiness or hyperactivity, and other behavioral disturbances. Parasomnias, such as sleep terrors, can become more frequent and severe with OSAS.

The sleep-wake pattern can also reveal if sleep-disordered breathing is affecting sleep continuity. Frequent nighttime awakenings may indicate disrupted sleep due to repetitive obstructive respiratory events. Difficulty waking in the morning, excessive sleep need (eg, 12 to 14 hours of sleep in a school-age child), and/or daily naps are often manifestations of poor sleep quality.

Findings on physical examination disclose many of the risk factors or clinical sequelae of OSAS (Table 29-1). Obesity, defined as a BMI > 95th percentile, has a strong association with OSAS. In adult men, neck circumference greater than 17 inches correlates with increased risk for OSAS; this measurement can be obtained in older children or adolescents. Elevated blood pressure is one of the cardiovascular consequences of untreated OSAS. Enlarged or edematous nasal turbinates often accompany visible mouth breathing. A high-arched hard palate, small posterior airway, and

Chidekel AS, ed. *Curbside Consultation in Pediatric Sleep Disorders: 49 Clinical Questions* (pp. 135-138)

Table 29-1

Physical Examination Features Associated With Obstructive Sleep Apnea Syndrome in Otherwise Healthy, Nonsyndromic Children

• Hypertension • Obesity • Increased neck circumference • Increased abdominal girth	• Mouth breathing • Swollen nasal turbinates • High-arched palate • Enlarged palatine tonsils

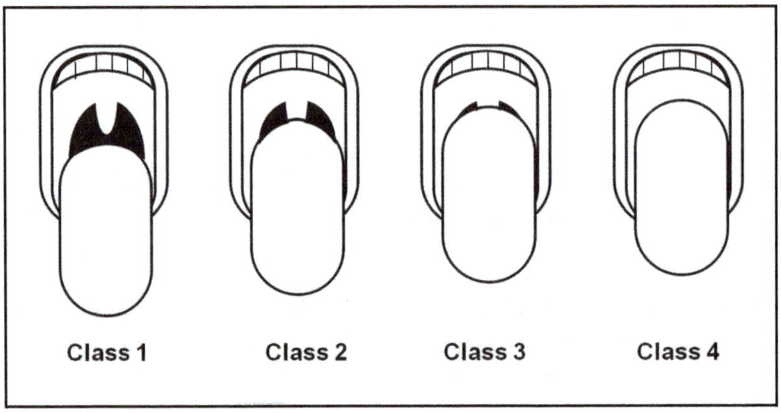

Figure 29-1. Modified Mallampati scoring: Class 1—tonsils, uvula, and soft palate visible; Class 2—hard and soft palate, top half of uvula, and upper portion of tonsils visible; Class 3—hard and soft palate and base of uvula visible; Class 4—hard palate visible.

tonsillar hypertrophy are oropharyngeal findings seen in children with OSAS. The Modified Mallampati classification used by anesthesiologists to evaluate the upper airway has also been used to determine the risk for OSAS. A Modified Mallampati class 3 or 4 airway is associated with a more difficult intubation and OSAS (Figure 29-1). A large body habitus and abdominal girth is another risk factor for sleep-disordered breathing.

When clinical evaluation suggests that a child may have OSAS, nocturnal polysomnography (PSG) performed in a sleep laboratory is the gold standard to confirm the diagnosis.[1] The parameters in these sleep studies include an electroencephalogram (EEG) to stage sleep and arousals, an electrooculogram (EOG) and chin electromyogram (EMG) to detect rapid eye movement (REM) sleep, an electrocardiogram (ECG), leg EMG to detect limb movements, oral-nasal airflow, thoracoabdominal effort, pulse oximetry, and body position. End tidal CO_2 and nasal pressure are additional parameters monitored in our pediatric sleep lab. An obstructive apnea episode is defined as minimal to no airflow despite continued thoracoabdominal respiratory effort for at least

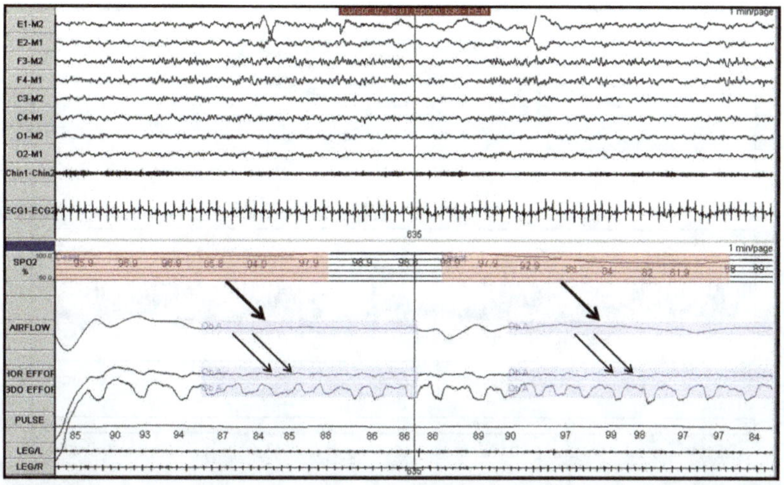

Figure 29-2. This diagram shows 2 obstructive apneas during a 1-minute interval during REM sleep in a polysomnogram. The bold arrow identifies the absence of airflow, and the double arrows show continued respiratory effort despite the absence of airflow.

2 respiratory cycles (Figure 29-2).[2] A hypopnea occurs when there is a ≥30% decrease in airflow for at least 2 respiratory cycles associated with ≥3% oxygen desaturation, an arousal or an awakening.[2] The apnea-hypopnea index (AHI) is the number of apneas and hypopneas per hour of sleep. In general, an obstructive AHI>1 is abnormal, although some sleep centers define pediatric OSAS as an AHI≥5. Associated comorbidities such as daytime sleepiness, behavioral problems, and hypertension may influence management when the AHI is between 1 and 5. A proposed pediatric OSAS severity scale based on AHI is shown in Table 29-2.[3] In general, frequent or sustained desaturations below 80% raise the OSAS severity classification.

If PSG in the sleep laboratory setting is not feasible, home nocturnal oximetry studies and ambulatory or unattended PSG are other diagnostic options. Abnormal overnight oximetry studies can accurately screen for pediatric OSAS (Figure 29-3); however, normal oximetry requires confirmation with PSG as children with OSAS often have frequent arousals, rather than desaturations, associated with their obstructive respiratory events. Research studies have shown that ambulatory PSGs may detect OSAS in older children with moderate OSA (AHI>5), but data are lacking regarding the value of these studies on a broad clinical scale. Based on the current American Academy of Pediatrics guidelines, nocturnal in-laboratory PSG continues to be the gold standard for diagnosing pediatric OSAS.[1]

Because of the health consequences associated with pediatric OSAS and the potential need for surgical treatment, it is essential to accurately diagnose pediatric OSAS using clinical judgment and diagnostic tools. Objective data not only diagnose OSAS, but also determine the severity of disease, which influences the urgency of intervention and postoperative management, as those with severe OSAS may require inpatient observation after surgery.

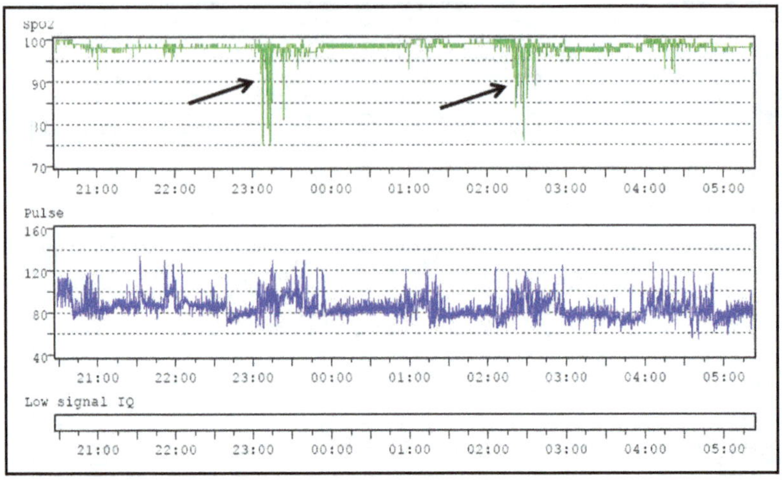

Figure 29-3. This overnight oximetry report shows clusters of desaturations (arrows), likely associated with obstructive respiratory events in a patient with a clinical history suggestive of OSAS.

Table 29-2

Pediatric Obstructive Sleep Apnea Syndrome Severity Scale

Mild OSA	Moderate OSA	Severe OSA
• AHI 2 to 5	• AHI 5 to 10	• AHI > 10

References

1. Marcus CL, Brooks LJ, Ward SD, et al. Technical report. Diagnosis and management of childhood obstructive sleep apnea syndrome. *Pediatrics*. 2012;130:e714-e755.
2. Iber C, Ancoli-Israel S, Chesson AL, Quan SF. *The AASM Manual for the Scoring of Sleep and Associated Events: Rules, Terminology, and Technical Specifications*. Westchester, IL: American Academy of Sleep Medicine; 2007.
3. Dayyat E, Kheirandish-Gozal L, Gozal D. Childhood obstructive sleep apnea: one or two distinct disease entities. *Sleep Med Clin*. 2007;2:433-444.

30 QUESTION

What Are the Nonrespiratory Consequences of Obstructive Sleep Apnea?

Holger Link, MD

Most of us think of obstructive sleep apnea as a disorder that mainly disrupts normal breathing during sleep. We picture a sleeping child that snores, has pauses in breathing, gasps for air and has intermittent drops in oxygen saturation associated with apnea events. Although this is a fairly typical presentation of sleep apnea, there are many children who snore or have noisy breathing without associated gasping or oxygen desaturations. Interestingly, even children with fairly mild obstructive sleep apnea can suffer adverse effects. Furthermore, there is not always a direct correlation between the severity of the sleep apnea, as measured by a sleep study, and the severity of adverse effects. The magnitude of the impairment depends not only on the severity of the sleep apnea, but it is also modified by such factors as sleep duration, environmental exposures, and genetically driven susceptibility. These factors interact in a complex fashion, which makes it difficult to precisely predict an individual child's impairment or risk of impairment in response to sleep apnea. In other words, there could be 2 children of the same age and gender with an identical severity of sleep apnea, but one of them would have no measurable negative effects and the other one would have significant learning and daytime problems. It is not yet entirely clear why some children are much more susceptible to the negative effects of sleep apnea.

Having recognized that children differ in their ability to tolerate sleep apnea, we can move on to discuss the specific consequences of obstructive sleep apnea. The 4 main systems affected are the brain, the metabolic, the cardiovascular, and the immune systems. These are summarized in Table 30-1.

Obstructive Sleep Apnea and the Brain

Obstructive sleep apnea can affect the brain in a variety of ways, depending on the severity of the apnea. Severe obstructive sleep apnea, with frequent obstructive events and oxygen desaturations, can lead to structural damage that includes the death of neurons and impaired synaptic connections. A major concern is that children with severe obstructive sleep apnea might sustain

Chidekel AS, ed. *Curbside Consultation in Pediatric Sleep Disorders: 49 Clinical Questions* (pp. 139-142)

Table 30-1

Examples of the Nonrespiratory Consequences of Obstructive Sleep Apnea Syndrome

Central Nervous System Consequences

- Hypoxic cellular injury
- Behavior problems
- Learning problems
- Excessive sleepiness
- Hyperactivity

Metabolic Consequences

- Increased insulin resistance
- Decreased growth hormone secretion
- Altered regulation of hunger and satiety

Cardiovascular Consequences

- Increased heart rate and vascular tone
- Systemic hypertension
- Pulmonary hypertension (rare)
- Cor pulmonale (rare)

Inflammatory Consequences

- Increased C-reactive protein levels
- Altered lymphocyte number and function

neuronal damage during a critical phase of brain development and that they are at high risk for persistent impairment, even after effective treatment of the sleep apnea.

One might think, on the other hand, that mild sleep apnea is a condition that we should not have to worry too much about. Unfortunately, that is not true. Even fairly mild obstructive sleep apnea without severe or frequent oxygen desaturations can lead to substantial behavioral or learning problems. This effect is thought to be mediated in part by frequent arousals that disrupt sleep continuity and quality. Arousals from sleep can be thought of as a protective response that prevents prolonged airway obstruction and hypoxia by briefly waking up the child and thereby increasing airway muscle tone leading to opening up of the airway. They occur, however, at the expense of diminished sleep quality.

One would expect that fatigue and sleepiness are universally present in children with sleep apnea as sleep quality is diminished. Remarkably, a significant number of children with sleep apnea do not display obvious fatigue and sleepiness. In addition, the symptoms will only become prominent in some children when demands on their performance increase—often, with the start of school. A child's inability to participate in class because of fatigue and sleepiness is a serious symptom that warrants further investigation.

Obstructive sleep apnea can impair learning and cognitive performance. Some children with obstructive sleep apnea have subtle learning problems that may only be revealed through formal standardized testing, whereas others have more overt problems that fairly readily come to the teacher's or parents' attention. It is important to be aware that performance and learning problems at school may be due to sleep apnea. If there is suspicion, one should take the time to ask the parents a few basic screening questions and evaluate the patient for risk factors. Is your child a quiet or noisy breather? Does your child's breathing during sleep look comfortable? Does your child sleep through the night? Is your child a restless sleeper? Does your child seem rested in the morning? In addition, one needs to take note of risk factors for obstructive sleep apnea, such as morbid obesity or a positive family history, and examine the patient's oropharynx for tonsil size and overall "roominess."

Disrupted sleep can lead to symptoms that mimic attention deficit hyperactivity disorder (ADHD) or attention deficit disorder (ADD). When encountering a new concern for inattention and hyperactivity or a formal diagnosis of ADHD or ADD, one should ask the simple screening questions stated previously and perform a quick examination of the patient's upper airway. Confirming a diagnosis of obstructive sleep apnea in these children can be very rewarding as treatment can result in the resolution or significant improvement of symptoms in some children.

Most of us know from our own experience that disrupted sleep can make the world look gloomier and our brains more irritable. Similar changes can occur in children with obstructive sleep apnea. They may display mood changes, irritability, or aggressive or defiant behavior. It is, therefore, prudent to explore the possibility of sleep apnea in a child with the onset of behavior problems.

Obstructive Sleep Apnea and Metabolism

Sound and restful sleep is not only important for our brain's normal function, but it also allows our body to rest, recharge, and recover. Obstructive sleep apnea disrupts the normal restorative functions of sleep and impacts important hormones that regulate glucose metabolism, somatic growth, and appetite.

Obstructive sleep apnea has been associated with negative changes in glucose metabolism. Patients with obstructive sleep apnea have increased insulin resistance and are at higher risk for diabetes. This effect is often magnified in obese children as they have a higher prevalence of obstructive sleep apnea and type 2 diabetes.

Growth hormone is secreted in a sleep-dependent fashion. Sleep disruption from sleep apnea has been shown to decrease growth hormone secretion. Conversely, treatment of sleep apnea has been shown to restore normal growth hormone secretion.

Restful sleep helps us maintain a normal appetite. Sleep disruption from obstructive sleep apnea can disturb the normal balance of hormones that regulate hunger and satiety. Patients with sleep apnea have lower levels of leptin and higher levels of ghrelin, with a net increase in appetite and risk for excessive weight gain.

Obstructive Sleep Apnea and the Heart

The cardiovascular system is usually in a more relaxed state during sleep as indicated by lower blood pressure, heart rate, and vascular tone. Obstructive sleep apnea interferes with the nocturnal rest period and can cause spikes in blood pressure, heart rate, and vascular tone. Fairly dramatic changes can be seen in children with severe sleep apnea during acute airway obstruction leading to a sensation of air hunger with intense activation of the sympathetic system. In rare cases, the sleep apnea is severe enough lead to pulmonary hypertension and cor pulmonale. However, even children with mild sleep apnea can have measurable changes in arterial blood pressure and increased vascular tone that are likely to be clinically significant over the course of several years.

Obstructive Sleep Apnea, Inflammation, and the Immune System

It has become increasingly clear over the last few years that sleep apnea is an inflammatory disorder.

The airway mucosa of patients with sleep apnea is chronically inflamed because of the nightly intermittent collapse of the airway and vibration of the pharyngeal tissues associated with snoring. However, in many patients, the inflammation is not confined to the upper airway, but is systemic. Increased levels of C-reactive protein and other inflammatory cytokines have been found in patients with sleep apnea. Although acute inflammation is an integral part of the body's defense system, chronic inflammation can have negative effects.

In addition to contributing to chronic inflammation, obstructive sleep apnea might also impair the normal function of the immune system. Recent studies have shown impairment in certain lymphocyte cell populations. The clinical significance of the findings is not yet entirely clear.

Summary

Obstructive sleep apnea has many effects that go well beyond the disruption of normal respiration during sleep. Patients with obesity and those with behavior problems are at higher risk for complications and should, therefore, be screened for obstructive sleep apnea and undergo a formal sleep study if there is a clinical suspicion.

Suggested Readings

Huang YS, Guilleminault C, Li HY, Yang CM, Wu YY, Chen NH. Attention-deficit/hyperactivity disorder with obstructive sleep apnea: a treatment outcome study. *Sleep Med.* 2007;8(1):18-30.

Kheirandish-Gozal L, Gozal D. Genotype-phenotype interactions in pediatric obstructive sleep apnea. *Respir Physiol Neurobiol.* 2013;13:S1569-9048.

Kim J, Hakim F, Kheirandish-Gozal L, Gozal D. Inflammatory pathways in children with insufficient or disordered sleep. *Respir Physiol Neurobiol.* 2011;178(3):465-474.

Landau YE, Bar-Yishay O, Greenberg-Dotan S, Goldbart AD, Tarasiuk A, Tal A. Impaired behavioral and neurocognitive function in preschool children with obstructive sleep apnea. *Pediatr Pulmonol.* 2012;47(2):180-188.

Nieminen P, Löppönen T, Tolonen U, Lanning P, Knip M, Löppönen H. Growth and biochemical markers of growth in children with snoring and obstructive sleep apnea. *Pediatrics.* 2002;109(4):e55.

Tan HL, Gozal D, Wang Y, et al. Neurocognitive and endothelial dysfunction in children with obstructive sleep apnea. *Pediatrics.* 2010;126(5):e1161-e1167.

QUESTION 31

What Are the Medical and Surgical Treatment Options for Pediatric Obstructive Sleep Apnea Syndrome?

Lewis J. Kass, MD

Because having obstructive sleep apnea (OSA) means that there is increased resistance to, or even absence of, airflow in the upper airway, the solution should be to decrease as much of that resistance as possible. A variety of techniques and strategies can be used to address increased upper airway resistance and pediatric OSA (Table 31-1) but, for the vast majority of children, this can be accomplished by surgical removal of both tonsils and adenoids. We used to quote that adenotonsillectomy fixed (cured) OSA completely in 90% of children. Those estimates have come down some in recent years,[1] but, given how many children respond so well to this procedure, it is one of the few areas in medicine in which a more invasive approach is chosen first over a less invasive approach. Some of the less invasive approaches that we'll discuss include the use of continuous positive airway pressure (CPAP), certain medications, weight loss, getting more sleep, the use of oral appliances, or even learning to play a wind instrument!

In 90% of cases in children, OSA is due to enlarged tonsils and adenoids (adenotonsillar hypertrophy). In a vast majority of lean and otherwise healthy kids, adenotonsillectomy (tonsillectomy and adenoidectomy [T&A]) is completely curative. When it comes to adenotonsillectomy, those of us in pediatric medicine usually advocate for the removal of both tonsils and adenoids. Often, a judgment call is made on the part of the surgeon to remove just one or the other depending on which tissue seems more likely to be the culprit. One can certainly understand a surgeon's conservative approach, given that removal of tonsils is a bloody surgery; is painful; and is associated with a longer recovery time, missed school time, and postoperative pain. On the other hand, a better fix usually occurs when both the tonsils and adenoids are removed. It was discovered a decade ago, via airway magnetic resonance imaging studies, that the area of greatest obstruction occurs at a level in the airway called the adenotonsillar overlap area[2]; hence, the need to remove both tonsils and adenoids. This pivotal imaging research that led to this understanding gave credence to what we have been recommending all along—namely, the complete removal of both tonsils and adenoids. A relatively new procedure that now seems in vogue is known as a *partial tonsillectomy*. There are

Chidekel AS, ed. *Curbside Consultation in Pediatric Sleep Disorders: 49 Clinical Questions* (pp. 143-146)

Table 31-1

An Overview of Treatment Options for Pediatric Obstructive Sleep Apnea Syndrome

Surgical Treatment • Adenotonsillectomy • Other specialized procedures
Positive Airway Pressure Therapy • CPAP • Bi-level positive airway pressure • Auto-titrating positive airway pressure
Medical Therapy • Intranasal corticosteroids • Montelukast • Antihistamine agents (possibly)
Nonmedical Therapy • Weight loss • Allergen avoidance • Environmental tobacco smoke avoidance • Playing a wind instrument

mixed reviews as to whether it really decreases postoperative discomfort and whether it results in the need to complete the procedure at a later date.

In children who do not have appreciable adenotonsillar tissue or for whom the ENT surgeon is hesitant to perform surgery, or for those for whom surgery did not work, CPAP is a very viable option. From the moment that you mention giving positive airway pressure with a snug-fitting mask connected to an air compressor every night, many parents will look at you sideways. Thus, working in a pediatric sleep center is important, where a family-centered approach can be taken. you will restore confidence when you explain that the CPAP titration sleep study will occur with your specialized pediatric CPAP technician and that, at the follow-up visit, you will have the pediatric sleep physician present and a home care vendor or respiratory therapist present capable of fitting a child with dozens of different pediatric masks and teach the use of the CPAP machine. When you follow that up with scheduling quarterly pediatric CPAP support groups (which we do at my pediatric sleep centers), you can generally promote excellent compliance. Finally, when you order state-of-the-art CPAP machines, namely the auto-titrating CPAP units, you optimize your chances of success. In one of my 2 pediatric centers, we start to titrate CPAP in children as young as 2.5 years of age. As you send the patient home with his or her machine, you want to instill into the family and the parent that some CPAP use is good, but more is better. I've found that with firm, but nonjudgmental encouragement, I wind up with more takers and improved adherence down the road.

Of course, there are going to be children that do not have very big tonsils or adenoids or those whom the ENT surgeon might deem too young to operate on. For these children, sometimes medication can be helpful. Medication aimed at shrinking adenotonsillar tissue and decreasing nasal congestion can often help decrease the resistance in the upper airway. These medications typically consist of using a nasal steroid with or without montelukast. Studies have shown that such a combination can at least help to downgrade the severity of a child's OSA.[3] Therefore, these anti-inflammatory and anti-allergic therapies are most useful in patients who have mild OSA. For children who have moderate-to-severe OSA, such a step probably does not change much in any appreciable way for a symptomatic child. However, for a baby and toddler, for whom growth may provide the ultimate cure for OSA, a medication-based approach can often help him or her bide his or her time until such growth occurs.

Oral appliances are another step occasionally used in children when T&A is not an option. Generally, these devices are designed to help pull the lower jaw forward. In so doing, they pull the tongue forward as well and may help decrease some of the upper airway obstruction when it might be due to the tongue falling back (posteriorly) in the oropharynx during sleep. Of all the treatment options for OSA, this is probably the one that is used least often. Oral appliances are generally most effective for patients with mild or positional OSA. A more important deterrent, though, is that dental sleep specialists are usually hesitant to manipulate the jaw until most of a child's growth is done.

Weight loss deserves mention. With obesity on the rise in children and adolescents, obesity is a growing source of OSA in the pediatric population.[4] Therefore, weight loss is always recommended but, unfortunately, is sometimes difficult to accomplish. It has been found, however, that there is a close link between obesity, metabolism, and obstructive sleep apnea.[5] It turns out that having OSA can lead to insulin resistance and subsequent obesity. It has also been shown that using CPAP in this situation improves metabolism and enhances weight loss—thus breaking the cycle of obesity → OSA → insulin resistance → worsening obesity → worsening OSA.

Regarding factors for obesity, it has also been found that disturbed nighttime sleep of any source can alter metabolism. Furthermore, not getting enough sleep (sleep restriction) has been associated with altered metabolism.[6] Because sleep restriction or sleep disturbance independent of OSA can alter metabolism, it highlights the importance of improving sleep quality (and quantity) to hopefully prevent getting into the cycle of obesity and OSA. It turns out our mothers were right—we need to get our sleep!

Finally, as bizarre or unconventional as it might sound, if no other options are available, or if a family is completely against CPAP, surgery, or medications, then it might be more desirable to describe the potential value of playing a wind instrument. For example, the didgeridoo, an ancient wind instrument that has been played by the aboriginal population in Australia for over 1500 years, has been found to improve symptoms of sleepiness and the apnea-hypopnea index in adults.[7] Theoretically, if a person's OSA is due to upper airway collapsibility, then playing a wind instrument is thought to prevent or ameliorate such collapse by strengthening and toning the airway musculature. It should be noted, however, that these findings have not been replicated in children. Furthermore, it is well known that a child's airway and the possible mechanisms of its collapsibility are different than an adults. Regardless, I have found that suggesting to a parent that playing a wind instrument could be potentially helpful (and certainly could not hurt) shows them you are open-minded and willing to discuss alternative options. This can only foster trust that may prove necessary in combating OSA down the road.

OSA is a significant problem in children and can have far-reaching consequences, ranging from irritability, poor school performance, displaying symptoms of attention deficit hyperactivity disorder, having nocturnal enuresis, and poor growth to having profound effects on heart, lung, and metabolic function. Children with OSA may appear chronically ill and certainly utilize health care resources significantly more frequently than children without OSA.[8] Therefore, it is vital to identify children with OSA and find a way to eliminate the obstruction, whether it is through surgery, CPAP, or a variety of the other options outlined previously.

References

1. Bhattacharjee R, Kheirandish-Gozal L, Spruyt K, et al. Adenotonsillectomy outcomes in treatment of obstructive sleep apnea in children: a multicenter retrospective study. *Am J Respir Crit Care Med.* 2010;182:676-683.
2. Arens R, McDonough JM, Corbin AM, et al. Upper airway size analysis by magnetic resonance imaging of children with obstructive sleep apnea syndrome. *Am J Respir Crit Care Med.* 2003;167(1):65-70.
3. Kheirandish L, Goldbart AD, Gozal D. Intranasal steroids and oral leukotriene modifier therapy in residual sleep-disordered breathing after tonsillectomy and adenoidectomy in children. *Pediatrics.* 2006;117(1):e61-e66.
4. Gozal D, Kheirandish-Gozal L. The obesity epidemic and disordered sleep during childhood and adolescence. *Adolesc Med State Art Rev.* 2010;21(3):480-490:viii-ix.
5. Nakra N, Bhargava S, Dzuira J, Caprio S, Bazzy-Asaad A. Sleep-disordered breathing in children with metabolic syndrome: the role of leptin and sympathetic nervous system activity and the effect of continuous positive airway pressure. *Pediatrics.* 2008;122(3):e634-e642.
6. Ju SY, Choi WS. Sleep duration and metabolic syndrome in adult populations: a meta-analysis of observational studies. *Nutr Diabetes.* 2013;3:e65.
7. Puhan MA, Suarez A, Lo Cascio C, Zahn A, Heitz M, Braendli O. Didgeridoo playing as alternative treatment for obstructive sleep apnea syndrome: randomized controlled trial. *BMJ.* 2006;332(7536):266-270.
8. Tarasiuk A, Greenberg-Dotan S, Simon-Tuval T, et al. Elevated morbidity and healthcare use in children with obstructive sleep apnea syndrome. *Am J Respir Crit Care Med.* 2007;175:55-61.

QUESTION 32

Is CPAP Therapy Used in Children?

Raj Padman, MD

Children with obstructive sleep apnea syndrome (OSAS) experience repeated episodes of partial or complete airway obstruction during sleep. This can result in drops in oxygen saturation, a rise in carbon dioxide levels, and sleep disruption. OSAS remains an underdiagnosed disorder and is a common cause of morbidity in approximately 2% of children. The prevalence of OSAS does not differ between the sexes during childhood. Documented comorbidities of OSAS in children include failure to thrive, as well as neurocognitive, cardiovascular, metabolic, and inflammatory sequelae. With this background knowledge, more children are being referred to sleep laboratories for polysomnography.

Anatomic narrowing and the neuromuscular tone of upper airway musculature determine the propensity for upper airway collapse during sleep. Increased resistance in the nasal compartment may relate to anatomic narrowing of the nasopharynx caused by allergic rhinitis, nasal turbinate hypertrophy, deviated nasal septum, and maxillary constriction. Adenoidal hypertrophy, palatal factors, tongue base collapse, macroglossia, posterior displacement of the mandible, and craniofacial syndromes cause narrowing of the oropharynx. Collapse or constriction in either of these anatomic locations, or both, can result in OSAS. Several medical conditions result in an increased risk for OSAS, including obesity, craniofacial disorders, neuromuscular disorders, sickle cell disease, premature birth, trisomy 21, and other genetic disorders. Adenotonsillar hypertrophy is the most common cause of OSAS in children aged 2 to 8 years. Adenotonsillectomy is the preferred treatment for most patients with OSAS. Sleep-related airway obstruction and quality of life measures improve in the majority of children postsurgery.

Persistent respiratory abnormalities may be seen in as many as 25% to 50% of children on postoperative polysomnography. Postoperative polysomnography is recommended in children with persistent symptoms, underlying conditions, or severe preoperative OSAS. Children with unresolved OSAS despite adenotonsillectomy, particularly those with abnormal craniofacial anatomy

Chidekel AS, ed. *Curbside Consultation in Pediatric Sleep Disorders: 49 Clinical Questions* (pp. 147-150)

or neuromuscular tone and obesity, may require additional treatment of persistent OSAS. These children are the primary candidates for long-term therapy with positive airway pressure (PAP) therapy. Nonsurgical treatment of sleep-related breathing disorders with PAP support has a role as a second-line therapy in pediatrics as opposed to in adults when it is first-line therapy.

The indications for use of PAP support while asleep include the following:

- Persistent obstructive sleep apnea despite adenotonsillectomy
- Patients not considered candidates for airway surgery
- Patients with complex sleep apnea
- Perioperative management of severe obstructive sleep apnea or obstructive sleep apnea complicated by pulmonary hypertension and cor pulmonale

PAP therapy can be continuous (CPAP) or bi-level (BiPAP). CPAP involves a continuous, but constant, level of positive airway pressure, whereas BiPAP consists of a higher inspiratory pressure and a lower airway pressure applied on exhalation. Applying positive pressure to the airway orifice mechanically stents the airway open. The usual negative inspiratory forces generated during breathing and that tend to collapse the airway are opposed, resulting in decreased work of breathing, improved lung volumes, and stabilization of oxygenation, as well as the restoration of sleep continuity and decreased sleep fragmentation.

The level of PAP needed to overcome obstructive sleep apnea and hypopnea, ameliorate snoring, and normalize gas exchange is achieved by an attended polysomnography, and this is safe and efficacious in children. PAP titration is ideally done by an experienced technologist after the initial diagnostic sleep study, allowing time for the patient and family to understand and accept the mask interface. Successful titration to final pressure involves resolution of snoring, apnea, hypopnea, arousal, and any gas exchange abnormality through multiple sleep stages in various body positions. In general, lower levels of CPAP are needed in pre-pubertal children. Adolescents appear to require similar levels of pressure as adults. Recurrent snoring and increased daytime sleepiness despite documented compliance indicates the need for a repeat sleep study to possibly adjust airway pressures. Significant changes in weight and age with growth can change the airway pressure requirements as well.

The specific nasal mask interface that is used needs to be documented and the introduction of smart cards in PAP devices has improved objective data regarding adherence and the success of therapy. In general, there are 3 types of mask interfaces employed in PAP therapy. Nasal pillows are the smallest and are essentially oversized nasal prongs that fit within the nares. Nasal masks fit over the entire nose (Figure 32-1) and full face masks cover both the mouth and the nose. Note that a patient wearing a full face mask must be able to remove the mask independently. Serial clinical follow up is essential to provide ongoing encouragement, education, and troubleshooting regarding the device and the patient interface. In addition, it can be anticipated that the mask size and optimal CPAP levels will change with growth.

The complications and recommendations to avoid PAP complications are as follows:

- Discomfort and skin irritation and redness related to pressure effect on the nasal bridge from a tight-fitting mask: Possible recommendations for addressing this problem may include using a different mask size or configuration or using nasal pillows. Using an occlusive dressing to protect the skin at the mask interface may prevent skin irritation.
- Eye irritation or conjunctival injection: The way to overcome this is to avoid leaks, and to reposition and refit the mask.

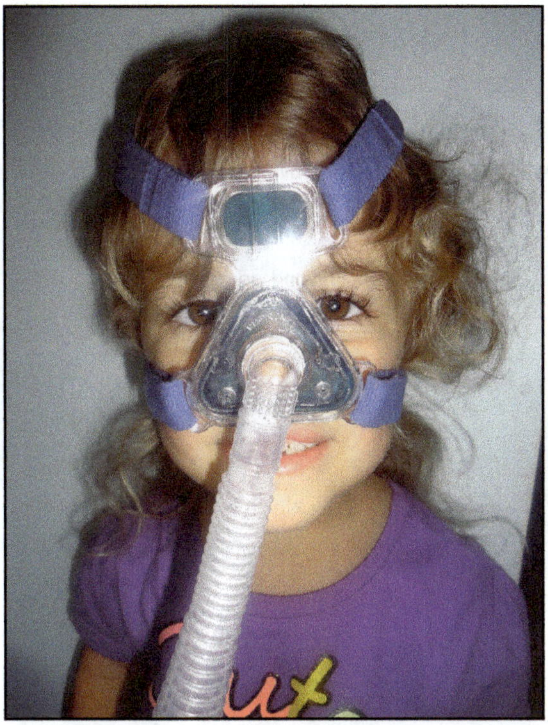

Figure 32-1. An example of a nasal mask for use with PAP therapy.

- Nasal congestion, nasal dryness, and irritation: The way to overcome this is to use heated humidification.
- Aerophagia/gastroesophageal reflux: The way to overcome this is to decrease the pressure.
- Mid-facial hypoplasia with long-term use: The way to overcome is to alternate mask types.
- Chest discomfort and pneumothorax: The way to avoid this is to decrease pressure.
- Compliance/adherence: Adherence remains an important issue. High dropout rate and suboptimal nightly use have been reported with PAP therapy in all ages. Most school-age children and adolescents who received dedicated education and follow-up were adherent to PAP therapy. Patients with higher baseline apnea-hypopnea indices and greater changes in apnea-hypopnea indices on PAP therapy were more likely to be adherent. Adherence was not associated with gender, race, age, or BMI.

Summary

PAP therapy is an important adjunctive modality for children of all ages with severe or persistent OSAS. PAP therapy physically stents open a collapsible upper airway, reducing apnea and hypopnea events, ameliorating snoring, and improving sleep quality. Attention to mask size and type enhances both patient comfort and acceptance of therapy, and ongoing follow-up is critical to both clinical efficacy and patient adherence.

Suggested Readings

American Thoracic Society. Indications and standards for use of nasal continuous positive airway pressure (CPAP) in sleep apnea syndromes. *Am Respir Crit Care Med*. 1994:150:1738-1745.

Chakravorty S, Frinder J. Positive airway pressure therapy in children. *Sleep Med Clin*. 2010;5:439-449.

Chediak A. Manual titration of positive airway pressure in patients with obstructive sleep apnea. *Sleep Med Clin*. 2009;4:443-453.

Harford KL, Jambhekar S, Com G, et al. Behaviorally based adherence program for pediatric patients treated with positive airway pressure. *Clin Child Pschol Psychiatry*. 2013;18(1):151-163.

Praud JP, Dorion D. Obstructive sleep disordered breathing in children: beyond adenotonsillectomy. *Pediatr Pulmonol*. 2008;43:837-843.

Uong E, Eppersion M, Bathon S, Jeffe D. Adherence to nasal positive airway pressure therapy among school-aged children and adolescents with obstructive sleep apnea syndrome. *Pediatrics*. 2007;5:120.

33 QUESTION

How Do I Best Evaluate the Snoring Child?

Ignacio E. Tapia, MD

Snoring, one of the symptoms of sleep-disordered breathing (SDB), is common in pediatrics. Caregivers report that approximately 7.5% of children snore as reported by caregivers.[1] Snoring and the obstructive sleep apnea syndrome (OSAS) are within the continuum of OSAS. The latter has been associated with significant morbidity when untreated, such as systemic and pulmonary hypertension, endothelial dysfunction, and neurobehavioral deficits, among others. Lately, developmental deficits have also been linked to snoring. A recent study including 249 children showed that children aged 3 years who snored more than 2 times per week during the past year had significantly higher reported hyperactivity, depression, and inattention compared to age-matched nonsnoring children.[2] Importantly, similar results have been reported in older children. In Germany, 69 children with primary snoring (PS) documented by a normal polysomnogram (PSG) were compared to children who never snored. Researchers reported that hyperactive, inattentive behavior, and daytime sleepiness were more frequently described in children with PS compared to never snorers.[3] Therefore, it is important to evaluate snoring children not only to rule out OSAS, but to diagnose and possibly prevent snoring associated morbidities as well.

Clinical Assessment

The first step in the evaluation of the snoring child is a detailed history and physical exam. Specifically, you should ask caregivers for the frequency and characteristics of snoring to rule out other causes of noisy breathing during sleep, such as stridor. A seasonal predominance of symptoms, for instance, could suggest allergic rhinitis. During the physical exam (Table 33-1), one should pay attention to the growth curve as obesity and, to a lesser extent, failure to thrive have been associated with OSAS. It is very important to perform a detailed exam of the head, looking for such craniofacial anomalies as micrognathia, retrognathia, and adenoidal facies; to examine the nose, looking for causes of nasal obstruction, such as deviated septum, polyps, and foreign bodies in younger children; to examine the oropharynx, evaluating for a modified Mallampati

Chidekel AS, ed. *Curbside Consultation in Pediatric Sleep Disorders: 49 Clinical Questions* (pp. 151-154)

Table 33-1

Physical Exam Findings

Growth chart	Obesity Failure to thrive
Head	Adenoidal facies Micrognathia Retrognathia Craniofacial anomalies
Nose	Deviated septum Polyps Foreign bodies
Oropharynx	Mallampati classification Tonsils size Tongue Size
Dental	Caries
Thorax	Pectus excavatum

classification of the upper airway, tonsils size, tongue size, and other indirect signs of mouth breathing, such as caries. Pectus excavatum could be present in children as a consequence of the negative pressure resulting from breathing against an occluded upper airway during the episodes of obstructive apnea.

Research has shown that parental report and physical examination have a weak association between objective snoring characteristics and the diagnosis of OSAS. This limitation is likely due, at least in part, to social factors, as parents who sleep close to their children may be more prone to listen to their snoring. In addition, the relaxation of the upper airway muscles during sleep may lead to anatomical changes that are not present during wakefulness.

Radiologic Assessment

A lateral neck radiograph is useful in the evaluation of the snoring child (Figure 33-1). The mouth should be closed (this may be challenging in younger children), and the head and neck hyperextended to provide a better view of the upper airway. This radiograph permits adequate estimation of the adenoidal pad and tonsillar size. Further, radiologic airway narrowing has been shown to increase the probability of OSAS on PSG.

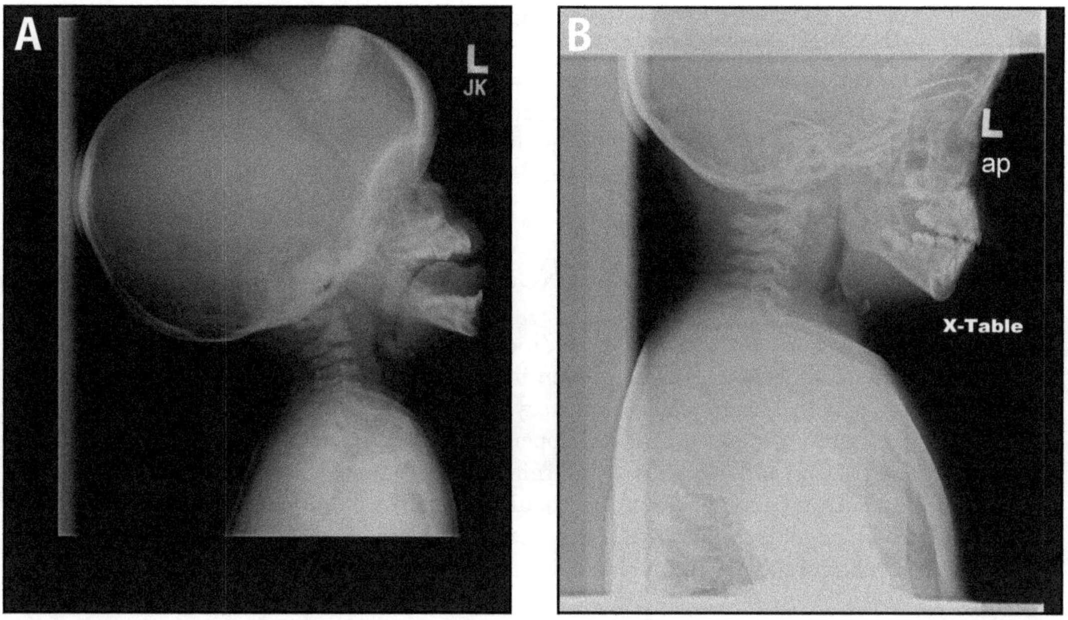

Figure 33-1. (A) Lateral neck radiograph of a child with achondroplasia. Note the frontal bossing and midface hypoplasia, which limit upper airway size and increase the risk of obstructive sleep apnea. (B) Lateral neck radiograph of a child with Down syndrome. Note the midface hypoplasia, which limits upper airway size and increases the risk of obstructive sleep apnea.

Endoscopy

Endoscopy provides a direct visualization of adenoidal tissue, palatine, and sublingual tonsils.

Nocturnal Oximetry

There are limited studies in children comparing nocturnal oximetry to PSG. These have shown inconclusive test results, poor sensitivity, and specificity. Therefore, they are not recommended for the study of the snoring child, as data resulting from these could be misleading. Normal oximetry does not rule out significant sleep-disordered breathing in an otherwise healthy child with normal pulmonary reserve.

Polysomnography

Nocturnal attended in-laboratory PSG is considered the gold standard to differentiate between PS and OSAS, as it provides a quantitative evaluation of breathing pattern during sleep.[4] Basically, a laboratory PSG records electroencephalographic, bilateral electrooculograms, chin electromyogram, limb movements, electrocardiogram, nasal pressure, airflow, end-tidal CO_2, oxyhemoglobin saturation, and chest wall and abdomen breathing movements data. In addition, many laboratories have infrared video recording capabilities that are extremely useful in the evaluation of artifacts. Thus, it is the most comprehensive tool in the evaluation of sleep.

Because a nocturnal attended in-laboratory PSG is expensive and not widely available, in-home unattended sleep studies—in other words, ambulatory PSG—have been developed. These studies provide less information as they usually record only cardiorespiratory data and there are no personnel to adjust loose leads or correct possible artifacts. There are few studies in children comparing ambulatory to in-laboratory PSG, but all of them were performed in older children and resulted in conflicting results. Therefore, they cannot be recommended at this point.

Summary and Recommendations

Snoring is common in children and, in addition to being a symptom of OSAS, it has been recently linked to neurobehavioral deficits even in the absence of OSAS. The evaluation of the snoring child starts with a comprehensive history and physical exam. A lateral neck radiograph is a useful tool to assess the patency of the upper airway, but the gold standard to differentiate between primary snoring and OSAS is an overnight in-laboratory polysomnogram. Because this test may not be available in many cities, one should refer those children with a high suspicion of OSAS—those with craniofacial anomalies or genetic syndromes, such as Down syndrome, achondroplasia, neurobehavioral deficits, obesity, kissing tonsils, and pectus excavatum.

References

1. Lumeng JC, Chervin RD. Epidemiology of pediatric obstructive sleep apnea. *Proc Am Thorac Soc.* 2008;5(2):242-252.
2. Beebe DW, Rausch J, Byars KC, Lanphear B, Yolton K. Persistent snoring in preschool children: predictors and behavioral and developmental correlates. *Pediatrics.* 2012;130(3):382-389.
3. Brockmann PE, Urschitz MS, Schlaud M, Poets CF. Primary snoring in school children: prevalence and neurocognitive impairments. *Sleep & Breathing.* 2012;16(1):23-29.
4. Marcus CL, Brooks LJ, Draper KA, et al. Diagnosis and management of childhood obstructive sleep apnea syndrome. *Pediatrics.* 2012;130(3):e714-e755.

QUESTION 34

What Are the Differences Between Pediatric and Adult Obstructive Sleep Apnea Syndrome?

Rocio Zeballos-Chavez, MD and Lynn A. D'Andrea, MD

Epidemiology

In nonobese and otherwise healthy children, the prevalence of obstructive sleep apnea syndrome (OSAS) ranges from 1% to 5%. Habitual snoring is common during childhood and affects approximately 10% of children aged 2 to 8 years; the frequency of snoring decreases after the age of 9 to 10 years. Boys and girls are equally affected by OSAS until adolescence, when it becomes more common in boys, which is similar to the adult pattern. The prevalence of OSAS is 6% to 9% in men and 3% to 4% in women—a ratio of approximately 2 to 3:1.

OSAS occurs more commonly among Black children and adults, compared with Whites of the same age groups. The incidence of OSAS is similar for Hispanic compared to White children.

Obesity confers an additional risk for sleep-disordered breathing in all races and both genders.

Pathophysiology

Upper airway patency is maintained by structures surrounding the upper airway, including cartilage and bony structures. In addition, airway patency is maintained by neural input to upper airway dilator muscles surrounding the upper airway. Abnormalities in any of these structures results in anatomic narrowing or collapse of the upper airway. In children, the most common cause of OSAS is adenotonsillar hypertrophy. Children with craniofacial anomalies (eg, Down syndrome) or neuromuscular disease (eg, Duchenne muscular dystrophy, cerebral palsy) are also at risk to develop sleep apnea. Obesity is a major risk factor for OSAS in both children and adults, although it is still a more common cause in adults.

Chidekel AS, ed. *Curbside Consultation in Pediatric Sleep Disorders: 49 Clinical Questions* (pp. 155-157)

Diagnosis

Clinical Symptoms

Snoring is the most frequent symptom that brings either a child or an adult to medical attention. Parents often describe the child as having paradoxical respiratory efforts ("belly breathing"), as well as being quite restless and sweaty during sleep. The child often positions him- or herself with the mouth open and the neck hyperextended back.

In regard to daytime symptoms, adults with OSAS frequently complain of daytime sleepiness, even falling asleep at their job or while driving a motor vehicle. Daytime sleepiness is a more ominous finding in children with OSAS, and they typically present with concerns for hyperactivity or difficulty with concentration at school. Several studies have shown an association with OSAS and children diagnosed with attention deficit hyperactivity disorder.

Physical Examination

In children with OSAS, the most prominent finding is adenotonsillar hypertrophy. Children with OSAS may be overweight, but most are of normal weight and a few are actually underweight, perhaps because of the increased work of breathing or fragmented sleep with resultant poor growth. Adults with OSAS often have associated hypertension; this is not as common a finding in children.

Polysomnography

Children with OSAS often have partial obstructive events rather than complete upper airway obstruction. The American Academy of Sleep Medicine has separate rules for scoring respiratory events in children. An obstructive apnea is scored if there is a ≥ 90% drop in airflow and respiratory efforts are present; the apnea meets criteria if it occurs for ≥ 2 breaths or 6 seconds. A hypopnea is scored if all of the following criteria are met:

- The airflow drops by ≥ 30%
- The event is associated with a 3% drop in oxygen saturation or is associated with an arousal
- The event lasts for ≥ 2 breaths or 6 seconds

The severity of OSAS, based on the apnea-hypopnea index (AHI), varies between children and adults (Table 34-1).

Sleep specialists who score and interpret pediatric sleep studies must be familiar with the differences in normal sleep architecture between children and adults. Sleep architecture is age-dependent with a maturational process occurring during the first decade of life. Children with OSAS often have normal sleep architecture with few arousals, whereas adults with OSAS have frequent arousals, as well as decreased delta and REM sleep.

Management

Surgical

Adenotonsillectomy is considered the primary treatment for children with OSAS and is generally considered curative. More recently, some studies have shown that up to 45% of children have residual OSAS following surgery, so clinical re-evaluation is important. Surgery is not the primary treatment option for adults with OSAS. Other more complex, secondary airway surgeries

Table 34-1

Differences in Obstructive Sleep Apnea Syndrome Severity in Children and Adults

Severity	*Children AHI Score*	*Adults AHI Score*
Mild OSAS	2 to 5	5 to 15
Moderate OSAS	>5 to 10	>15 to 30
Severe OSAS	>10	>30

AHI = Apnea-hypopnea index.

employed by otolaryngologists to optimize airway patency in both children and adults include nasal turbinate reduction, lingual tonsillectomy, palatopharyngoplasty, hyoid suspension, genioglossal advancement, and rapid maxillary expansion.

Medical

Noninvasive ventilation using positive airway pressure (PAP) is the primary treatment for adults with OSAS. PAP therapy is used for children with persistent OSAS, despite surgical management, or for children who are not candidates for surgical intervention. It is used as a temporizing measure for children with severe OSAS who are awaiting surgery. Unfortunately, PAP therapy is becoming increasingly common for children with morbid obesity and OSAS.

Oral appliances are indicated for adults with mild to moderate OSAS. They are used much less commonly in children because of the concern of damage to, or the disruption of, the underlying growing facial skeletal structures.

Other interventions to decrease upper airway inflammation or swelling include anti-inflammatory medications, such as topical nasal steroids or leukotriene inhibitors. These therapies can be used in both children and adults with mild OSAS. Finally, weight reduction or positional therapy can be recommended for both children and adults with OSAS. Depending on the age of the child and severity of the obesity, some weight management plans for children encourage them to maintain their weight while "growing into it" over time (ie, growing taller) rather than following an absolute weight-reduction program.

Suggested Readings

Berry RB, Brooks R, Gamaldo CE, et al. *The AASM Manual for the Scoring of Sleep and Associated Events. Rules, Terminology and Technical Specifications*. Darien, IL: American Academy of Sleep Medicine; 2012:39-47.

Bonuck K, Freeman K, Chervin RD, Xu L. Sleep-disordered breathing in a population-based cohort: behavioral outcomes at 4 and 7 years. *Pediatrics*. 2012;129:e857-e865.

Kaditis A, Kheirandish-Gozal L, Gozal D. Algorithm for the diagnosis and treatment of pediatric OSA: a proposal of two pediatric sleep centers. *Sleep Med*. 2012;13:217-227.

Marcus CL, Brooks LJ, Draper KA, et al. Clinical practice guideline: diagnosis and management of childhood obstructive sleep apnea syndrome. *Pediatrics*. 2012;130(3):576-584.

Young T, Palta M, Dempsey J, et al. Burden of sleep apnea: rationale, design, and major findings of the Wisconsin Sleep Cohort study. *WMJ*. 2009;108(5):246-249.

SECTION VII

SLEEP AND MEDICAL CONDITIONS AND GENETIC DISORDERS

QUESTION 35

What Are Some of the More Common Genetic Syndromes That Are Associated With Sleep-Disordered Breathing?

Vandna Passi, MD

Sleep patterns are intricately related to our genetic make-up, body structure, muscle strength, and neuronal wiring. Therefore, we often see sleep-disordered breathing in individuals with the protean genetic diseases that affect this delicate framework so dramatically. Minute molecular changes in our DNA can lead to obvious phenotypical changes that interfere with the respiratory and neurological equilibriums needed to achieve ideal sleep quality. We will discuss some of these disorders in this chapter and also look at treatment options to promote normal ventilation and adequate restful sleep in people who have sleep-disordered breathing related to these underlying genetic disorders. Some of these conditions are also described in Question 28, and specific craniofacial syndromes that affect sleep are discussed in Question 36. Tables 35-1 and 35-2 list some additional syndromes that the practitioner should recognize as being related to sleep and breathing, and the reader is referred to recent practice guidelines or review articles listed in the "Suggested Readings" section at the end of this chapter for additional detail.

Duchenne Muscular Dystrophy

Duchenne muscular dystrophy (DMD) is an X-linked recessive genetic disorder that affects the male children of female carriers of the abnormal gene. This is one example of many congenital (or acquired) myopathies that will impact respiration during sleep due to muscle weakness. The dystrophin gene is disrupted in DMD and is critical in the formation of the protein that provides structural stability to muscle cell membranes. This progressive disease results in muscle hypertrophy and eventual weakness due to muscle cell death. Around the teenage years, most children with DMD become wheelchair-bound. Concurrently, patterns of restrictive lung disease become evident and are manifested by weak cough, poor airway clearance, and insufficient achievement of tidal volume in the supine position due to diaphragmatic and accessory muscle weakness,

Chidekel AS, ed. *Curbside Consultation in Pediatric Sleep Disorders: 49 Clinical Questions* (pp. 161-166)

Table 35-1

Selected Genetic and Craniofacial Syndromes Associated With Snoring and Obstructive Sleep Apnea

• Achondroplasia • Apert syndrome • Arthrogryposis • Beckwith-Wiedemann syndrome • Campomelic dysplasia • Crouzon syndrome • Down syndrome • Hunter's syndrome	• Klippel-Feil syndrome • Marfan syndrome • Pfeiffer syndrome • Rubinstein-Taybi syndrome • Stickler syndrome • Treacher Collins syndrome • Velocardiofacial syndrome

Table 35-2

Selected Genetic Conditions and Syndromes Associated With Abnormal Control of Breathing

- Arnold-Chiari malformation
- Congenital central hypoventilation syndrome (CCHS)
- Joubert syndrome
- Rett syndrome
- Spina bifida

ultimately causing nocturnal hypoventilation and possibly upper airway obstruction as well. Thus, while sleeping, it is more difficult to maintain a tidal volume sufficient for adequate oxygenation because conscious control of respiration and gravity are not assisting the airway dilating and respiratory muscles in the same way as when an individual is awake and upright. Pulmonary function testing can alert the physician objectively when the vital capacity is less than 40% or when daytime hypoventilation becomes apparent. Modalities such as continuous positive airway pressure (CPAP) or bi-level positive airway pressure (BiPAP) are often initiated after a sleep study is performed to objectively document obstructive sleep apnea syndrome, nocturnal hypoventilation, or even respiratory insufficiency. These devices provide adequate inspiratory and/or expiratory distending pressures to maintain ventilation while asleep.

Prader-Willi Syndrome

Prader-Willi syndrome (PWS) is a rare genetic disorder in which there is a microdeletion of some genes inherited from the paternal side of chromosome 15 (q 11-13). Manifestations of this disease include hypotonia, failure to thrive in infancy, obesity as an older child, and learning disabilities. PWS can be associated with sleep-related comorbidities, including OSA and secondary narcolepsy. Children with PWS should be evaluated with a polysomnogram regularly to assess for sleep-disordered breathing, and polysomnography is specifically recommended around the initiation of human growth hormone therapy as well. Risk factors for developing sleep-disordered breathing in children with PWS include the following:

- Significant obesity
- Asthma
- Symptoms consistent with OSA, such as frequent nocturnal awakenings and/or daytime somnolence
- The initiation of growth hormone therapy

If a child is going for a procedure involving sedation or general anesthesia, it is recommended that he or she have a polysomnogram to avoid complications from sedation. For children who are found to have OSA, CPAP or BiPAP and weight reduction are the mainstays for therapy, and sometimes behavioral modifications are necessary for both of these therapies to be successful. Cataplexy, which is commonly seen in narcolepsy, is defined as a sudden loss of muscle tone that can last for a few seconds and can often be induced by emotion, such as laughter or crying. This can be seen in 16% to 23% of patients with PWS. These individuals may also experience frequent daytime somnolence and difficulty awakening, much like what is seen in narcolepsy. The mechanism underlying the connection between these 2 disorders has not been determined; however, there is some overlap in the symptoms of both these disease states. It is hypothesized that hypothalamic dysfunction may play a role in manifesting these symptoms in PWS, but conclusive evidence is yet to be established.

Congenital Central Hypoventilation Syndrome

Congenital central hypoventilation syndrome (CCHS) is a very rare disorder that affects 1 in 200,000 live births. It can be inherited by autosomal dominant pattern; however, over 90% of cases result from *de novo* mutations in the PHOX2B gene with no evidence of any family history. It is also important to note that about 5% to 10% of people affected by CCHS have parents with somatic mosaicism of the gene and that parental genetic testing should be discussed and offered in the context of genetic counseling at the time of a new diagnosis. CCHS affects neural development because the protein made from the gene PHOX2B is involved in neuronal formation and migration specifically within the autonomic nervous system. The autonomic nervous system is involved in many functions, one of which includes the central drive for breathing appropriately. State-dependent hypoventilation is the clinical hallmark of this disorder and can vary in severity depending on the severity of the genetic mutation in the PHOX2B gene. All patients with CCHS demonstrate hypoventilation during sleep that causes cyanosis and, despite inadequate ventilation, the brain is not alerted to awaken or augment respiration. Therefore, these individuals suffer from hypercarbia and hypoxia. If this is not addressed with adequate respiratory support, these children are at risk of suffering neurological injury or dying. The suggested modalities of treatment include tracheostomy placement and invasive mechanical mechanical ventilation only at night, although some children with more severe forms of CCHS require full-time ventilatory support. Children

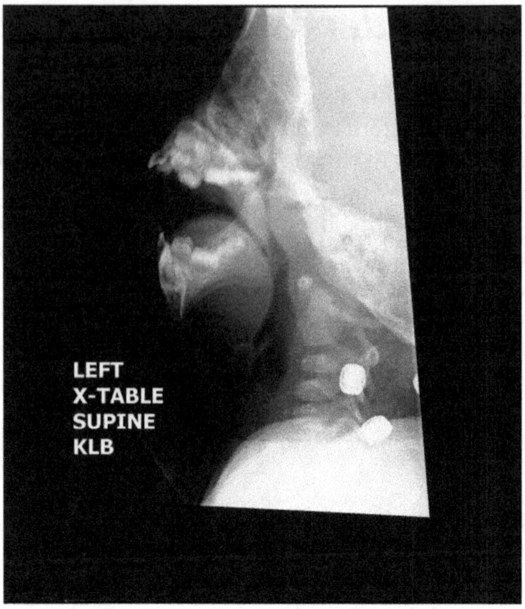

Figure 35-1. Lateral neck radiograph of a toddler with campomelic dysplasia revealing midface hypoplasia, micrognathia, and adenoidal hypertrophy.

with CCHS who require support only during sleep can be transitioned to nocturnal noninvasive positive pressure ventilation with a back-up rate later in childhood. CCHS is a complex disorder with additional systemic manifestations, a complete description of which is beyond the scope of this brief introduction to the clinical syndrome.

Skeletal Dysplasia Syndromes

Skeletal dysplasia syndromes are a group of diverse disorders that affect the growth and development of bones and cartilage. Most are autosomal dominant disorders caused by various genes that are involved with the growth and development of collagen and bone. Achondroplasia, campomelic dysplasia (Figure 35-1) and spondyloepiphyseal dysplasia congenita (SED) are 3 examples of such skeletal dysplasia syndromes. In achondroplasia, the gene affected codes for fibroblast growth factor receptor 3 (FGFR3). It is believed that abnormal FGFR3 activity results in abnormal bone growth. In campomelic dysplasia, the affected gene is called SOX9 (sex determining region-Y box gene), which codes for a protein that is critical during embryogenesis to the development of the skeletal and reproductive systems. SED is caused by mutations in the COL2A1 gene, which is responsible for a protein that makes type II collagen that is found in cartilage and allows for bones to develop normally. Each of these skeletal dysplasia syndromes causes various degrees of abnormalities in the formation of the skull and facial bones, along with abnormal growth and compliance of the chest cage. Abnormalities of the skull and facial bones can increase the risk of both central and obstructive sleep apnea and, because of a narrow chest wall, children may often experience difficulty ventilating, especially while asleep, because of restrictive lung disease. Another factor, particularly in infants or toddlers with SED, is tracheomalacia, or softening of the airway cartilage, that can contribute to airway obstruction as well. Despite their genetic commonalities, individual skeletal dysplasia syndromes can vary in severity, and some children do not need invasive interventions and are able to maintain adequate ventilation despite these opposing factors mentioned previously. Other times, children may need some nocturnal support with supplemental oxygen, CPAP, or BiPAP—or even invasive mechanical ventilation—until they have grown enough to establish adequate chest wall growth and strength to maintain adequate ventilation and oxygenation.

Rett Syndrome

Rett syndrome is a rare genetic disorder affecting the MECP2 gene located on the X chromosome. Other gene mutations have also been linked to the disease. It is a neurodegenerative disorder that affects social, motor, and intellectual development. Females are primarily affected with Rett syndrome. Clinical features of the disease include microcephaly, repetitive movements (particularly involving the hands and rocking motions), impaired communication, breathing abnormalities during wakefulness and sleep, loss of developmental milestones, bruxism, and cognitive dysfunction. Breathing abnormalities witnessed in this disease process vary in how they manifest. While awake, these children may display all or some of the following: hypoventilation, central apnea, episodic hyperventilation, air swallowing, and significant breath-holding. These variations in breathing patterns can lead to hypocarbia or hypercarbia depending on what the child is manifesting. Whether the child is hyperventilating vs hypoventilating or breath-holding, respectively, can affect the carbon dioxide level. While asleep, children with Rett syndrome can experience central apneas and/or hypoventilation due to OSA leading to hypercarbia. Families should be instructed to watch out for pauses in breathing during sleep because these may not be as common or obvious as breathing irregularities while awake. If any pauses or evidence of upper airway obstruction such as snoring are noted, a polysomnogram is recommended to evaluate this further.

Trisomies 13, 18, and 21

Trisomies 13, 18, and 21 occur when there is nondisjunction of one of these chromosomes during meiosis. Trisomy 13 results in Patau syndrome and manifests as physical deformities, including cleft palate, hypotonia, microphthalmia, and intellectual disabilities, as well as heart, brain, and spinal cord defects. Trisomy 18 is called *Edwards syndrome* and results in similar physical defects, along with rocker bottom feet, clenched or deformed hands, and feeding difficulties. Unless treated aggressively, children with either of these have a low rate of survival past the first year of life. The biggest complexities in these children that contribute to sleep issues mainly consist of hypotonia, oropharyngeal insufficiency, and cleft palate. These issues lead to frequent obstructive events and they will often need positive pressure support to alleviate that obstruction while asleep. Children with Trisomy 21 or Down syndrome have features of macroglossia, short stature, hypotonia, intellectual disability, simian crease, and upslanting eyes. The combination of a narrowed oropharynx with macroglossia and hypotonia cause obstructive sleep apnea to be very prevalent in this population. As these children grow older, some of them will develop obesity, which makes the risk of developing OSA more significant. Because there are behavioral and communicative difficulties in introducing an apparatus such as CPAP or BiPAP to these individuals, dietary modifications and nocturnal low-flow oxygen are also suggested as therapies. With patient, intensive family support and desensitization, however, PAP therapies can be implemented in select cases. Nevertheless, serial polysomnography and periodic monitoring of gas exchange during wakefulness is recommended in this population to assess for developing OSA. Historical information about snoring, daytime somnolence, and pauses in breathing while asleep are important to discern during outpatient evaluations.

Suggested Readings

Baumann CR, Bassetti CL, Scammell TE. *Narcolepsy: Pathophysiology, Diagnosis, and Treatment.* New York: Springer Verlag; 2011.

Birnkrant DJ, Bushby KM, Amin RS, et al. The respiratory management of patients with Duchenne muscular dystrophy: a DMD Care Considerations Working Group specialty article. *Pediatr Pulmonol.* 2010;45(8):739-748.

Bull MJ, the Committee on Genetics. Clinical report—health supervision for children with Down syndrome. *Pediatrics.* 2011;128(2):393-406.

Deal CL, Tony M, Höybye C, Allen DB, Tauber M, Christiansen JS. 2011 growth hormone in Prader-Willi Syndrome Clinical Care Guidelines workshop participants. Growth Hormone Research Society workshop summary: consensus guidelines for recombinant human growth hormone therapy in Prader-Willi syndrome. *J Clin Endocrinol Metab.* 2013;98(6):e1072-e1087.

Trotter TL, Hall JG, and the Committee on Genetics. Health supervision for children with achondroplasia. *Pediatrics.* 2005;116(3):771-783.Weese-Mayer DE, Berry-Kravis EM, Ceccherini I, Keens TG, Loghmanee DA, Trang H. ATS Congenital Central Hypoventilation Syndrome Subcommittee. An official ATS clinical policy statement: Congenital central hypoventilation syndrome: genetic basis, diagnosis, and management. *Am J Respir Crit Care Med.* 2010;181(6):626-644.

U.S. National Library of Medicine. Description of "Congenital Central Hypoventilation Syndrome" on "Genetics Home Reference" page, http://ghr.nlm.nih.gov/condition/congenital-central-hypoventilation-syndrome. Accessed September 16, 2015.

Young D, Nagarajan L. Sleep problems in Rett syndrome. *Brain Dev.* 2007;20(10):609-616.

36 QUESTION

What Are Some of the More Common Craniofacial Syndromes That Are Associated With Sleep-Disordered Breathing?

Vandna Passi, MD

Facial structure and the genes involved in creating the architecture of the face are vital in our daily function—not only in routine activities during wakefulness, such as eating, speaking and breathing, but also when we sleep. The positioning of the facial muscles, organs, and nerves will provide support to the upper airway to ensure adequate airway patency and ventilation while asleep, and particularly during supine sleep. Children who have disorders that either disrupt the process of facial formation from proceeding correctly in fetal development or halt its progression in infancy and early childhood are at high risk of developing abnormal sleep quality, sleep-disordered breathing, and obstructive sleep apnea syndrome. Children with these disorders often need interventions over many years medically and surgically to correct the disrupted process and to augment airway function.

Pierre Robin Sequence

Pierre Robin sequence (PRS) involves facial malformations, including micrognathia, glossoptosis, and cleft palate. This combination of defects produces a malformed, small oropharynx that puts babies and children with this disorder at risk for upper airway obstruction and obstructive sleep apnea. The tongue often is displaced backwards and can partially or completely occlude the airway, particularly when an infant or child is supine. The small mouth and chin make the effect of the occlusion more likely to occur and causes sleep-disordered breathing. It is recommended that infants with PRS and severe glossoptosis sleep prone or even lie on their side. In our practice, we monitor these infants with pulse oximetry chronically to ensure that oxygenation is maintained at an acceptable level.

To augment the size of the airway, certain surgical techniques have been implemented, including glossopexy, a tongue-adhesion procedure that will attach the tongue to the bottom of the

Chidekel AS, ed. *Curbside Consultation in Pediatric Sleep Disorders: 49 Clinical Questions* (pp. 167-170)

mouth so that it does not roll back. When infants get older, they become eligible to undergo a jaw extraction surgery so that the airway increases in diameter, although some centers are using this technique in neonates. Children with PRS often have respiratory insufficiency, especially during sleep, and will sometimes need positive pressure support or even tracheotomy until they have grown enough to have these more definitive procedures performed. The cleft palate is usually repaired at around 1 year of age.

Cleft palate becomes an important topic of discussion at this point because it is not only seen in this disorder, but can be seen in various other syndromes and sequences and also as an entity by itself from multifactorial genetic influences. Cleft palate can be complete or partial and can involve only the hard palate or both the hard and soft palates. It involves the disruption of the palatal musculature and tissue, causing an abnormal opening that can put the infant at risk for aspiration, nasopharyngeal reflux, and poor weight gain due to poor feeding skills. Cleft lip is sometimes associated with this deformity as well. It has been shown that infants with cleft palate are prone to developing obstructive sleep apnea (OSA). The small oropharynx that may be related to the cleft deformity is causative in the ensuing sleep apnea, and surgical intervention, such as a tonsillectomy, often helps treat OSA after diagnosis with a sleep study. In fact, as in otherwise healthy children, a tonsillectomy and adenoidectomy is often curative for sleep-disordered breathing. Repeat sleep study is recommended to ensure resolution of symptoms after sufficient healing time from surgery.

Treacher Collins Syndrome

Treacher Collins syndrome (TCS) is a rare autosomal dominant disorder distinguished by craniofacial deformities due to the absence of—or because of malformed—facial bones. The gene mutation involved in most of these individuals is the TCOF1 gene, and microdeletions or missense mutations cause variable phenotypic features, depending on what aspect of the gene is defective. Approximately 40% of patients with TCS have inherited disease, while the remaining individuals are affected by *de novo* mutations. The protein from this gene mutation is called *treacle* and it aids in accurate neural crest cell migration, particularly in the first and second pharyngeal arches, which play a major role in the development and formation of the craniofacial structures.

OSA in TCS can result from facial malformations, particularly because of nasal and pharyngeal involvement of the upper airway in this disorder. Polysomnography establishes the need for airway or positive pressure interventions; however, the underlying facial anomalies need to be corrected surgically when the child is old enough for reconstruction. Often, bone grafts from other parts of the body, such as the ribs, are used for skeletal reconstruction of the facial features to help these children with normal orofacial function.

Apert Syndrome and Crouzon Syndrome

Apert syndrome—also referred to as *acrocephalosyndactyly syndrome*—is an autosomal dominant disorder that affects males and females equally. In a population, 1 in 200,000 is affected and most cases are due to *de novo* mutations. The gene involved in this disorder is the fibroblast growth factor 2 gene on chromosome 10, causing a mutational defect in the protein that induces apoptosis in certain cells to not take place, thus causing malformations of the hands, feet, and face. The disorder affects the first branchial arch or pharyngeal arch that is responsible for the formation of the maxilla and mandible and the structures supporting them. The clinical features of the disease include craniosynostosis further affecting the shape and structure of the face, as well as syndactyly, which causes webbing of the fingers and toes.

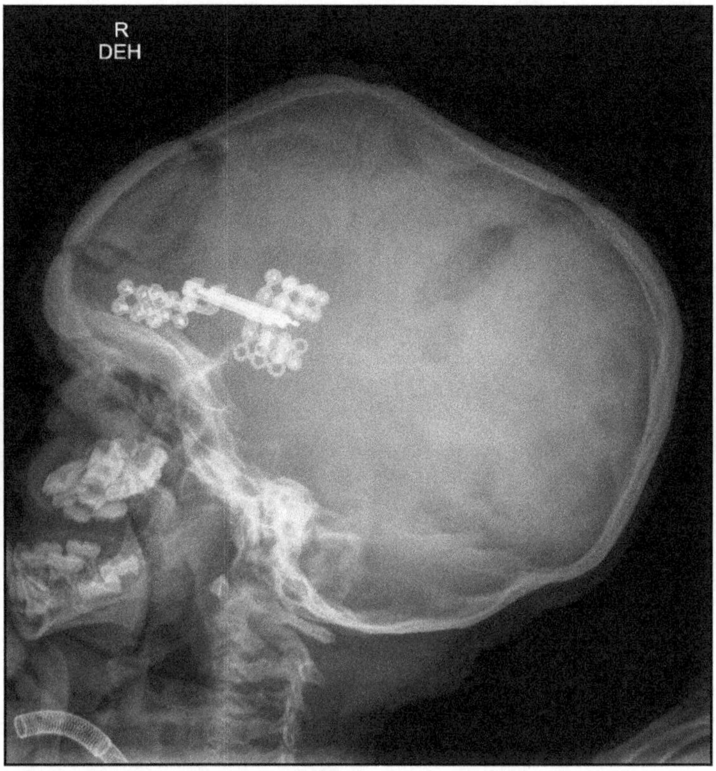

Figure 36-1. Lateral neck and skull radiograph of a patient with Apert syndrome requiring long-term tracheotomy due to upper airway obstruction. Note the extreme midface hypoplasia.

Briefly, craniosynostosis involves premature fusion of the cranial sutures, which affects the shape of the skull and influences the direction in which the brain will grow and expand over the first year of life. Features of craniosynostosis include a high prominent forehead and a flattened area in the posterior area of the head. This causes abnormal facial features, including wide-spaced eyes and low-set ears. Brachycephaly is the most common growth pattern of the skull that occurs with premature closure of the coronal suture.

Crouzon syndrome presents very similarly to Apert syndrome and involves the same gene and protein defect. The clinical features of Crouzon syndrome are more varied in that someone with this disorder may have very mild midface hypoplastic features to very severe clinical manifestations, whereas children with Apert syndrome often have very similar characteristics. The facial features in Crouzon syndrome affect the eyes more profoundly, and these children may present with exophthalmos, strabismus, and a beaked-nose appearance due to prominent orbital bones.

Facial deformities that result from Apert syndrome (Figure 36-1) include crowding of the teeth, protrusion of the mandibular area due to narrowing of the palate, and a high-arched palate. This leads to a narrow oropharyngeal area that is prone to insufficiency during sleep and causes airway obstruction. These children will have OSA due to facial deformities and may need support with noninvasive or invasive positive pressure ventilation via facemask or tracheostomy tube, depending on the severity of sleep apnea and airway function. Because of the underlying abnormal facial features, it is important to consider using an appropriate interface if CPAP or BiPAP is needed to ensure proper delivery of positive pressure.

Summary

Although any of the many and varied craniofacial syndromes can lead to upper airway narrowing, dysfunction, and obstructive sleep apnea syndrome, Pierre Robin sequence and Apert, Crouzon, and Treacher Collins syndromes are classic examples that should be known to any pediatric practitioner. In addition to routine pediatric care, craniofacial and sleep medicine specialists will be important members of the health care team for children with these complex disorders. Frequent discussions of sleep and breathing, as well as regular polysomnographic testing, will be important in their successful management.

Suggested Readings

Anderson IW, Sedaghat AR, McGinley BM, et al. Prevalence and severity of obstructive sleep apnea and snoring in infants with Pierre Robin sequence. *Cleft Palate Craniofac J.* 2011;48(5)614-618.

Dreissen C, Joosten KF, Bannink N, et al. How does obstructive sleep apnoea evolve in syndromic craniosynostosis? A prospective cohort study. *Arch Dis Child.* 2013;98:538-543.

Robison JG, Otteson TD. Increased prevalence of obstructive sleep apnea in patients with cleft palate. *Arch Otolaryngology Head Neck Surg.* 2011;137(3):269-274.

QUESTION 37

WHAT DO I NEED TO KNOW ABOUT SLEEP AND BREATHING IN CHILDREN WITH UNDERLYING LUNG DISEASES?

Michael Blechner, MD and Anita Bhandari, MD

Effective sleep is extremely important in our daily lives and contributes significantly to proper growth and development in children. Sleep comprises almost half of a child's life, and inadequate sleep is associated with multiple health concerns, including a higher incidence of attention deficit disorder (ADD) and obesity, to name a couple. Therefore, it is important to know who is at risk for sleep-disordered breathing (SDB). Understanding the physiology of breathing and chest wall mechanics forms the basis for SDB with underlying lung disease.

In normal conditions, sleep offers less effective breathing than while awake. Minute ventilation (with a decrease in respiratory rate and tidal volume) and functional residual capacity are decreased, while airway resistance is increased. During sleep, there is a decrease in upper airway and intercostal muscle activity, which further leads to less efficient breathing during sleep. These effects are greater in rapid eye movement (REM) sleep and magnified in children, compared to adults, since children sleep longer than adults and REM sleep comprises a greater percentage of sleep in childhood.

When thinking about children with SDB secondary to underlying lung disease, the 3 most common lung diseases are as follows:

1. Asthma
2. Cystic fibrosis (CF)
3. Bronchopulmonary dysplasia (BPD)

Other conditions that are much less common, such as neuromuscular disease and chest wall abnormalities, can cause a restrictive lung disease without lung parenchymal or airway disease components.

Chidekel AS, ed. *Curbside Consultation in Pediatric Sleep Disorders: 49 Clinical Questions* (pp. 171-174)

Asthma

Asthma is the most common lung disease encountered in children. Asthma has long been thought to interfere with a child's sleep. Many causes of SDB in asthma have been put forth, including persistent airway inflammation, poor airway clearance, and circadian rhythm abnormalities of cortisol and histamine. In patients with severe asthma exacerbations, an impaired peripheral chemoreceptor function and a poor respiratory load perception have been implicated to cause further worsening of nocturnal hypoxemia as well.

The majority of research studies on patients with asthma and SDB use snoring as a marker for the presence of SDB as sleep studies are often difficult and expensive to obtain. Not only is asthma a risk factor for habitual snoring, but habitual snorers are twice as likely to have asthma compared to children who did not snore. Wheezing and nocturnal cough have also been found to occur more commonly in patients who snore compared to those who do not. In fact, cough and persistent wheeze have been reported to be the strongest predictors of SDB when patients have undergone home monitoring for SDB. There may be an association between asthma severity and SDB as well. A recent study shows asthma patients with SDB are 3 times more likely to have severe asthma as compared to those who did not have SDB.[1]

Patients with more frequent asthma symptoms report a greater daytime sleepiness and tiredness as compared to children with less frequent asthma symptoms and those with no asthma symptoms. Greater incidence of sleep problems in those with more frequent asthma symptoms without a significant difference in sleep parameters, including sleep latency, nighttime awakenings, and time in bed, suggests a significant relationship between asthma symptom control and sleep.[2] It is quite obvious that asthma and SDB are comorbid conditions and that the presence of one often worsens the symptoms of the other. National Heart, Lung, and Blood Institute guidelines for management of asthma recommend that one look for SDB in patients with unstable and difficult-to-control asthma.

Management

Management is largely supportive. Optimization and adherence to asthma therapy should be considered. Improvement in asthma control in patients with obstructive sleep apnea (OSA) and tonsillo-adenoidal hypertrophy postsurgery has been reported.[1]

Cystic Fibrosis

Sleep disturbances seem to be common and occur early in the course of CF. Changes in upper airway and respiratory function during sleep will further accentuate gas exchange abnormalities that may exist in patients with CF. Although CF patients often report poor quality of sleep, it does not predict nocturnal gas exchange. Furthermore, in children with clinically stable CF, nocturnal oxygen saturation is lower than those with no CF.[3] CF children with normal forced expiratory volume in 1 second (FEV_1)have been shown to have a significantly lower sleep efficiency as compared to controls and a progressive drop in sleep efficiency with a decline in FEV_1.[4] As CF lung disease progresses, SDB worsens. Patients with severe CF lung disease report lower sleep efficiency, a greater degree of sleep fragmentation, and lower oxygen saturations. This sleep fragmentation may well be related to nocturnal coughing from impaired mucociliary clearance, among other factors. Although we know that patients with CF have sleep disturbances, there are no clear guidelines for obtaining a polysomnogram (PSG). In our practice, we usually order a PSG if the patient has clinical symptoms of SDB, has baseline daytime hypoxia, and/or is going to need noninvasive ventilation (NIV) for chronic respiratory failure.

Management

Management includes aggressive airway clearance to improve mucociliary clearance and, thus, minimize ventilation-perfusion mismatch. Aggressive management of an intercurrent pulmonary exacerbation has been shown to improve oxygen saturations in patients who develop low nocturnal oxygen saturations when sick. For patients with CF and SDB, treatment options include supplemental nocturnal oxygen, which improves nocturnal oxygenation, increases time spent in REM sleep, and shortens sleep latency. Also, use of supplemental oxygen in patients with severe lung disease results in better tolerance of exercise and school/work attendance. Supplemental oxygen administration, however, carries the risk of worse hypercapnia. Fortunately, this increase in CO_2 has been found to have little clinical consequence. NIV has been used in patients with CF, in addition to oxygen, to help with gas exchange during sleep, especially in patients with moderate and severe lung disease. Although NIV is less commonly used in CF as compared to other chronic diseases, it does help by decreasing respiratory muscle workload and the work of breathing. This results in improved gas exchange when used along with supplemental oxygen, as compared to supplemental oxygen alone.

Bronchopulmonary Dysplasia

Children with BPD have poor respiratory reserve and are at risk for greater respiratory morbidity throughout childhood when compared to their full-term peers. Prematurity has been identified as a risk factor for development of OSA later in life, but the presence of SDB in former premature babies is an area of research that has been overlooked. Often, clinical symptoms such as failure to thrive, prolonged need for oxygen, and development of pulmonary hypertension in former premature infants is attributed to the underlying lung disease rather than to SDB. Data from PSGs obtained for the purpose of weaning oxygen, evaluating adequacy of ventilatory support, or to rule out obstructive sleep apnea show that outpatient respiratory rates and oxygen saturations were not predictive of oxygen saturation nadir and respiratory disturbance index observed on PSG. However, infants with BPD had lower oxygen saturations and a higher respiratory disturbance index—findings that are not entirely surprising. Central apnea events and bradycardia events on PSG did correlate with patients' respiratory rates recorded outpatient. The authors attribute this to impaired alveolarization and altered pulmonary mechanics; both findings are well documented in former premature babies with BPD. In patients who had more than one study, there was a decrease in the number of apnea events and respiratory disturbance index on subsequent studies, suggesting that SDB improves as these children age.[5]

Management

Management is based on the cause of SDB. If a patient has OSA and adenotonsillar hypertrophy, then surgical treatment should be considered. In those where the predominant finding is that of central apnea, consideration may be given to prolonged oxygen supplementation. Assessment of nutritional status and optimization of medical treatment of underlying lung disease, including diuretic therapy, should be considered.

Neuromuscular Diseases

Patients with an underlying neuromuscular disease, such as Duchenne muscular dystrophy (DMD) and spinal muscular atrophy (SMA), develop a progressive restrictive lung disease. DMD is the most common myopathy affecting respiratory function. Children with DMD, starting as early as 2 years of age, have progressive muscle weakness that initially affects proximal muscles and eventually involves respiratory muscles. Patients will have nocturnal hypoventilation or hypopnea, especially in REM phase. This is thought to be related to a pre-existing muscle weakness, which is further accentuated in REM phase of sleep. This, along with weakness of the upper airway causing OSA, results in hypercapnia and hypoxemia, which both cause frequent arousals, resulting in poor sleep efficiency. SMA leads to respiratory insufficiency and subsequent failure through progressive muscle weakness due to the degeneration of anterior horn cells of the spinal cord. There are several types of SMA based on age of onset and degree of impairment. Those with significant respiratory muscle weakness (Type 1 and some with Type 2) will often develop an ineffective cough, sleep apnea, and nocturnal hypoventilation, much like patients with DMD.

Management

Supportive care, including aggressive airway clearance, will help with the quality of sleep by decreasing arousals from frequent cough. On the other hand, pulmonary function tests obtained during daytime are not a good reflection of nocturnal gas exchange, so a detailed history to rule out SDB is crucial. It is recommended that a PSG be obtained if a patient has a FEV1 < 40%, a base excess of 4 mmol/L, $P_aCO_2 > 54$, and low daytime oxygen saturations.[6] NIV is recommended in those with SDB. As neuromuscular weakness progresses and the patient is not able to remain off NIV for a prolonged period of time, placement of tracheostomy and positive pressure ventilation may be needed.

Summary

Underlying obstructive and restrictive lung diseases may accentuate and exacerbate SDB in children. Early diagnosis and aggressive management of both underlying lung disease and SDB are crucial to improving quality of life, and decrease mortality and morbidity.

References

1. Ross K. Sleep-disordered breathing and childhood asthma: clinical implications. *Curr Opin Pulm Med.* 2013;19:79-83.
2. Van Mammen A, Wiiga AH, Poatma DS, et al. Sleep in children with asthma: results of the PIAMA study. *Eur Respir J.* 2013;41:832-837.
3. Van der Giessen L, Bakker M, Joosten K, Hop W, Tiddens H. Nocturnal oxygen saturation in children with stable cystic fibrosis. *Pediatr Pulmonol.* 2012;47(11):1123-1130.
4. Amin R, Bean J, Burklow K, Jeffries J. The relationship between sleep disturbance and pulmonary function in stable pediatric cystic fibrosis patients. *Chest.* 2003;128(3):1357-1363.
5. McGrath-Morrow SA, Ryan T, McGinley BM, Okelo SO, Sterni LM, Collaco JM. Polysomnography in preterm infants and children with chronic lung disease. *Pediatr Pulmonol.* 2012;47(2):172-179.
6. Arens R, Mazumdar H. Sleep, sleep disordered breathing, and nocturnal hypoventilation in children with neuromuscular diseases. *Paediatr Resp Rev.* 2010;11(1):24-30.

38

QUESTION

What Is the Impact of Obesity on Sleep?

Ambika Shenoy, MD

As health care providers for children, we commonly associate sleep-disordered breathing (SDB) with adenotonsillar hypertrophy. However, obesity is also a significant risk factor for SDB and disturbed sleep. Obese children experience more snoring at nighttime. Families often will describe other symptoms of SDB, including frequent nocturnal awakenings, restlessness, and witnessed pauses in breathing overnight. These symptoms interrupt sleep and cause daytime somnolence, fatigue, deteriorating school performance, and inattentiveness or ability to focus in class. Screening children who are overweight is particularly important because obesity and its associated sleep sequelae may negatively impact future growth and development. A provider should feel comfortable with identifying children at risk for SDB and sleep disruption. Furthermore, medically complex children with symptoms of SDB and sleep disruption, including those with obesity, should be referred to a pediatric sleep center for testing and treatment to mitigate negative effects on health.

Effects of Obesity on Respiratory Function

Obesity is defined as a body mass index (BMI) ≥ 95%, compared with children the same age and gender.[1] It is characterized by increased adipose tissue throughout the body. Deposition of adipose tissue on the waistline, chest, and neck negatively impacts respiratory mechanics and respiratory function. Abdominal adiposity may impair diaphragmatic excursion, while thoracic adiposity causes further "mass loading" of the chest wall. These changes require increased energy expenditure and effort to maintain respiration in obese individuals. As a result, obese patients typically exhibit a more rapid, shallow breathing pattern.

In addition, obese patients undergoing pulmonary function tests (PFTs) demonstrate several abnormalities that increase the risk for gas exchange abnormalities. Decreased functional residual capacity and reductions in expiratory reserve volume contributes to further abnormalities of gas exchange by reducing the oxygen reserves of the lung. There are also reports of increased airway

Chidekel AS, ed. *Curbside Consultation in Pediatric Sleep Disorders: 49 Clinical Questions* (pp. 175-178)

resistance and lower airway obstruction described with obesity. Diffusion impairment is also described, but this remains controversial as some studies suggest that diffusion capacity is preserved or increased in obese individuals.[2]

In children, the distribution of body fat rather than BMI may be a better predictor of abnormalities in sleep. For example, abdominal adiposity (measured by waist circumference) may correlate more with sleep-disordered breathing compared with such traditional measurements as BMI.[3] In sleep, the deposition of adipose tissue in the neck and posterior pharyngeal structures reduces the diameter of the upper airway and leads to partial airway obstruction. Taken together, providers must consider alterations in pulmonary function, airway adiposity, and adenotonsillar hypertrophy as contributors to SDB in obese patients. Suggested studies for evaluating SDB include polysomnogram (PSG) and measurements of pulmonary function (if clinically indicated) such as the following:

- Spirometry pre- and postbronchodilator administration (to assess for evidence of reversible airflow obstruction
- Body plethysmography (to assess lung volumes for the presence of either restrictive or obstructive lung disease)
- Measurements of diffusion capacity
- Airways resistance

These additional tests can be completed in conjunction with a pediatric pulmonologist or sleep center.

Causes of Sleep-Disordered Breathing in Obese Children

The PSG remains the test of choice to evaluate sleep staging, gas exchange, and respiratory pattern. One-third to almost a half of obese children undergoing screening for SDB will have an abnormal PSG.[4] A third of these patients will show moderate to severe abnormalities.[5] The most common disorders described are obstructive sleep apnea (OSA) and obesity hypoventilation syndrome, also known as Pickwickian syndrome. Other genetic disorders, such as Prader-Willi syndrome or rapid-onset obesity with hypothalamic dysfunction, hypoventilation, and autonomic dysregulation (ROHHAD) syndrome, may also present with obesity and symptoms of SDB or sleep disruption.[6] However, these illnesses are rare and typically present with additional specific clinical findings.

OSA syndrome is a common sleep disorder seen in children. The clinical manifestations, diagnosis, and treatment of OSA are discussed at length elsewhere within this book. Obesity is a significant risk factor for OSA and it is most commonly reported on PSG in overweight children. Symptoms are the result of altered pulmonary mechanics in combination with upper airway obstruction, possibly from adenotonsillar hypertrophy and deposition of adipose tissue in the neck and pharyngeal structures.[7] Obese children are at risk for the same sequelae of OSA as children with normal BMI. However, in obese children, it is difficult to differentiate the effects of being overweight from OSA because both may independently contribute to long-term complications.

A recent review article on the diagnosis and management of OSA describes the complications of OSA and addresses how obesity may contribute to their development.[8] For example, obese children may lack the normal "nocturnal dipping" of blood pressure during sleep. Furthermore, children with obesity are at risk for hypertension throughout the day and night. The presence of hypertension in the setting of sleep disturbance is an indication to pursue further testing.[9] Obese children also describe mood disturbances and behavioral difficulties. These are common entities

Table 38-1

Diagnostic Features of Obesity Hypoventilation Syndrome

- Obesity BMI > 30 kg/m^2
- Awake hypercapnia
- Absence of another cause of hypoventilation
- Sleep study reveals hypoventilation during sleep (with or without comorbid sleep apnea)

also described in children with OSA. Additional sequelae of untreated OSA include pulmonary hypertension, cor pulmonale, and cognitive delay.

Children with OSA and obesity are treated similarly to those with a normal BMI. Adenotonsillectomy is suggested if the child is a surgical candidate. Children with obesity undergoing surgery should be hospitalized and monitored postoperatively based on severity of OSA noted and other abnormalities of pulmonary function described. If significant abnormalities of gas exchange were seen preoperatively, follow-up PSG within a few weeks to months of surgery is suggested to ensure that signs/symptoms have resolved.[9] If they persist, or if the child is not deemed a surgical candidate, then he or she will benefit from initiation and titration of positive airway pressure (PAP). Weight loss should always be encouraged, as decreases in weight are associated with some improvement in nocturnal symptoms.

Obesity hypoventilation syndrome (OHS) is another insidious process that is difficult to differentiate from OSA based solely on symptoms of SDB described in clinic. Diagnostic features are listed in Table 38-1. In contrast to OSA, obese individuals without other known causes of hypoventilation demonstrate chronic hypercapnia, and possibly hypoxia, during the daytime and overnight while asleep. The exact pathophysiology of OHS is unknown; however, it is believed to occur in obese patients as a result of complex interactions between sleep-disordered breathing, impaired respiratory mechanics, and abnormalities of central respiratory control. This includes decreased ventilatory drive and altered central chemoreceptor sensitivity.[10] On PSG, the brainstem responses to acute changes or elevations in carbon dioxide are blunted in the presence of chronic hypercapnia. The presence of leptin-resistance in obesity may also represent an additional mechanism contributing to dysregulated central control of ventilation, but this requires further investigation.[10] If left untreated, patients with OHS are at risk for developing pulmonary hypertension, cor pulmonale, and other sequelae of obesity, including metabolic syndrome, hypertension, and stroke.

The diagnosis of OHS is made by establishing the presence of SDB and hypoventilation overnight on PSG, in addition to objective daytime measurements of elevated P_aCO_2. To evaluate OHS in obese children, the following tests may also be helpful:

- Pulse oximetry
- Capnometry (if available)
- Complete blood count (to assess for evidence of erythrocytosis from chronic hypoxemia)
- Electrolytes
- Arterial blood gas

Elevated serum bicarbonate in conjunction with normal pH and increased P_aCO_2 suggests metabolic compensation for chronic hypoventilation. Remember that hypercapnia will be missed if only pulse oximetry is measured in clinic!

Treatment of OHS is aimed at minimizing abnormalities of gas exchange and correcting abnormalities of central respiratory control. Weight loss should always be encouraged as part of treatment as it is associated with improvement in these entities. Similarly to OSA, adenotonsillectomy is suggested if the child has evidence of adenotonsillar hypertrophy and is a surgical candidate. Postoperatively, children should be hospitalized and monitored closely overnight due to dysregulation of respiratory control. Although it may take weeks to see improvement in the central response to hypercapnea, it is strongly recommended that PSG be repeated within a few months of surgery to ensure abnormalities of gas exchange have improved. If persistent deviations are found or the child is not a surgical candidate, they will benefit from initiation and titration of noninvasive positive pressure ventilation. Treatment with bi-level positive airway pressure is therapeutic for obese children with OHS. Adherence to PAP remains a concern. PAP should be initiated and titrated in a controlled setting rather than in the home environment. Children with OHS may depend more on hypoxic-mediated respiratory drive. Consequently, supplemental oxygen alone as a treatment for OSA or OHS is not recommended as this may exacerbate hypoventilation.

Summary

Obesity is an important risk factor for SDB and sleep disruption that requires regular screening and referral for further assessment. If left untreated, sequelae of untreated SDB associated with obesity can have detrimental effects on childhood growth and development. Weight loss, combined with surgical or medical interventions, is strongly suggested to treat OSA and OHS.

References

1. Barlow SE. Expert committee recommendations regarding the prevention, assessment, and treatment of child and adolescent overweight and obesity: summary report. *Pediatrics*. 2007;120(Suppl4):S164-192.
2. Salome CM, King GG, Berend N. Physiology of obesity and effects on lung function. *J Appl Physiol*. 2010;108(1):206-211.
3. Carotenuto M, Bruno O, Santori N, et al. Waist circumference predicts the occurrence of sleep-disordered breathing in obese children and adolescents: a questionnaire-based study. *Sleep Med*. 2006;7(4):357-361.
4. Marcus C. Evaluation of pulmonary function and polysomnography in obese children and adolescents. *Pediatric Pulmonology*. 1996;21:176-183.
5. Fiorino EK, Brooks LJ. Obesity and respiratory diseases in childhood. *Clin Chest Med*. 2009;30(3):601-608.
6. Ize-Ludlow D, Gray JA, Sperling MA, et al. Rapid-onset obesity with hypothalamic dysfunction, hypoventilation, and autonomic dysregulation presenting in childhood. *Pediatrics*. 2007;120(1):e179-e188.
7. Tauman RG. Obstructive sleep apnea syndrome in children. *Expert Reviews in Respiratory Medicine*. 2011;5(3):425-440.
8. Marcus CL, Brooks LJ, Davidson Ward S., et al. Diagnosis and management of childhood obstructive sleep apnea syndrome. *Pediatrics*. 2012;130(3):e714-e755.
9. Wise MS et al. Executive summary of respiratory indications for polysomnography in children: an evidence-based review. *Sleep*. 2011;34(3):389-398AW.
10. Piper AJ, Grunstein RR (2011) Obesity hypoventilation syndrome: mechanisms and management. *Am J Respir Crit Care Med* 2011;183(3):292-298.

QUESTION 39

What Is Known About the Relationship Between Sleep and Attention Deficit Hyperactivity Disorder?

Marianne C. San Antonio, DO and Rhonda Walter, MD

Attention Deficit Hyperactivity Disorder

Attention deficit hyperactivity disorder (ADHD) is a chronic neurobehavioral disorder associated with dopamine dysregulation in the prefrontal cortex of the brain marked by difficulties with executive functioning skills. These skills involve tasks such as sustaining attention, impulse control, time management, multitasking, and control of activity level. ADHD is diagnosed when a child has had marked impairment in attention and/or hyperactivity/impulsivity beginning before the age of 7 years that results in impairment in functioning across the home and school settings. These symptoms should not be due to other conditions that may impair a child's ability to concentrate, such as depression, anxiety, mania, psychosis, thyroid disease, substance use, or sleep impairments.[1] The relationship between ADHD and sleep is complex. It has been found that many children with ADHD have difficulties with sleep and that many children with sleep difficulties have behaviors that can look like ADHD, such as hyperactivity, inattention, irritability, difficulty focusing on tasks, and difficulty with peer interactions.[2] Both ADHD and sleep problems are common. Based on data collected by the CDC, the percentage of children diagnosed with ADHD in the United States ranges from 5.6% to 15.9%.[3] It has been reported that 25% to 50% of children with ADHD have sleep difficulties, including sleep-disordered breathing and periodic limb movements during sleep.[4] The percentage of children currently taking medication to treat ADHD in the United States ranges from 1.2% to 9.5%.[3] These medications may include stimulant and nonstimulant medications. Many families also turn to complimentary and alternative treatments that the practitioner should be aware of and which may also impact sleep.

Chidekel AS, ed. *Curbside Consultation in Pediatric Sleep Disorders: 49 Clinical Questions* (pp. 179-181)

Sleep and Attention Deficit Hyperactivity Disorder

Associated sleep dysregulations seen in children with ADHD can include excessive motor-driven activity, not shutting down to go to sleep, difficulty following family-based sleep rules, and attending to routine. Providers should also consider the possible impact of medications on the sleep cycle itself—either the direct effect of a stimulant or the rebound that can occur when medications wear off. Sleep quality can clearly impact daytime behavior. Certain mental health conditions and medications that may be used for ADHD can also impact a child's ability to sleep well. Children with ADHD are often reported to have difficulty with sleep initiation as they have difficulty calming down to go to sleep and following bedtime routines. Long-acting stimulant medications taken to treat ADHD can contribute to difficulties with sleep initiation. ADHD is commonly comorbid with anxiety disorders and mood disorders, which can disrupt sleep. Finally, in teenagers with ADHD, problems with drug and alcohol use can also impact sleep.

Snoring is 3 times more common in children with ADHD,[2] and children with snoring or sleep apnea are more likely to have some ADHD symptoms than children without these sleep disorders.[2] It has also been reported that many children with obstructive sleep apnea due to enlarged tonsils, who also have symptoms of ADHD, have improvement of their ADHD symptoms after a tonsillectomy.[5] This suggests that improving the quality of a child's sleep improves symptoms of inattention, hyperactivity, and impulsivity. It has also been shown that increasing the amount of sleep a child gets per night improves daytime behavior and decreasing the amount of sleep a child gets per night worsens daytime behavior.[6] Low ferritin levels can lead to periodic limb movements in sleep (PLMS), which can also disrupt sleep, and full-blown restless legs syndrome (RLS), like ADHD, has been correlated with low brain dopamine levels, indicating a possible common causal pathway.[2] RLS and PLMS are discussed in detail in Question 24.

Diagnosis and Management

ADHD is diagnosed based on history taken from parents, children, and teachers to understand a child's behavior at home and at school. It is treated through behavior modification at home and at school to teach executive functioning skills and by medications which decrease the core ADHD symptoms of inattention, hyperactivity, and impulsivity. When evaluating for ADHD, it is important to take a careful sleep history. This should include questions about breathing during sleep, sleep environment, bedtime routines, sleep duration, and peacefulness, as well as the timing and quality of sleep. In addition to asking about sleep, providers should also inquire about other mental health issues that can disrupt sleep, such as anxiety and mood disorders, and should screen teenagers for drug and alcohol use. Should any of these screening questions be positive, further evaluation should be done to diagnose and treat sleep and other mental health disorders before treating for ADHD.

Environmental, behavioral, and pharmacological contributors to sleep disturbance in children with ADHD should be considered and targeted for treatment (Table 39-1). Providers should ask about snoring, limb movements, and symptoms of RLS, and may want to check a ferritin level if a child is suspected to have RLS (a ferritin level of < 50 mcg/mL may indicate the need for treatment). One should consider ordering a sleep study in a child who snores and has other risk factors for obstructive sleep apnea.

Children diagnosed with ADHD should also be counseled on the importance of good sleep hygiene. This includes keeping a regular bedtime routine, consistent limit setting and consequences, and freedom from distraction (not watching television, playing video games, or listening to loud music in bed). Clinicians should also monitor sleep in children on longer-acting stimulant medications (especially those with duration of action greater than 8 hours or in children younger

Table 39-1

Sleep Management in Children With ADHD

Environmental	*Behavioral*	*Pharmacologic*
• Remove TV/video games from bedroom • Avoid loud music • Keep bedroom cool and dark	• Have a consistent nightly bedtime routine • Have a consistent bedtime	• Monitor long-acting stimulant effects • Consider shorter acting stimulants • Consider non-stimulants (alpha-agonists)

than 6 years of age). Consideration should be given to using shorter-acting formulations if sleep initiation difficulties occur. Using nonstimulant medications, such as the alpha-agonists, as an alternative or adjunct treatment to stimulants, can help with both the treatment of ADHD and difficulties with sleep initiation. There is currently insufficient evidence to support the use of complementary and alternative medicines, such as diets or vitamin supplements, for the treatment of ADHD.

References

1. American Psychiatric Association. *Diagnostic and Statistical Manual of Mental Disorders: DSM-IV* (4th ed., text rev.). Washington, DC: American Psychiatric Association; 2000.
2. Owens JA. A clinical overview of sleep and attention-deficit/hyperactivity disorder in children and adolescents. *Journal of the Canadian Academy of Child and Adolescent Psychiatry/Journal de l'Academie canadienne de psychiatrie de l'enfant et de l'adolescent.* 2009;18(2):92-102.
3. Centers for Disease Control and Prevention Attention-Deficit/Hyperactivity Disease website. http://www.cdc.gov/ncbddd/adhd/index.html. Accessed June 15, 2015.
4. Chervin RD, Archbold KH. Hyperactivity and polysomnographic findings in children evaluated for sleep-disordered breathing. *Sleep.* 2001;24(3):313-320.
5. Chervin RD, Ruzicka DL, Giordani BJ, et al. Sleep-disordered breathing, behavior, and cognition in children before and after adenotonsillectomy. *Pediatrics.* 2006;117(4):e769-e778.
6. Gruber R, Cassoff J, Frenette S, Wiebe S, Carrier J. Impact of sleep extension and restriction on children's emotional lability and impulsivity. *Pediatrics.* 2012;130(5):e1155-e1161.

QUESTION 40

What Are Some of the Other Medical Conditions That Can Affect Sleep?

Jennifer Shroff Pendley, PhD and Aaron S. Chidekel, MD

Children with acute and chronic medical conditions frequently experience significant difficulties with sleep. Hospitalizations, pain, stress of illness, medication, and disease processes can affect the quantity and quality of sleep that, in turn, can have a profound effect on the child's overall health and quality of life and also on caregiver well being. During hospitalizations, sleep can be impacted by pain, hallway noise, light, blood pressure and temperature checks, and overall unease from being in an unfamiliar environment. In addition, pain and sleep have a bidirectional relationship in that pain can disrupt sleep cycles, and sleep deficits are associated with increased perceptions of pain. Furthermore, medications and disease processes can impact both the quality and quantity of sleep and, while examples of these conditions range from the mild to the complex, respiratory symptoms often predominate in their contribution to sleep disruption (Table 40-1).

Rhinitis is a common and multifactorial pediatric condition, with an incidence of up to 40% in some series, which can have a major impact on the quality and quantity of sleep in childhood. Rhinitis may be allergic or nonallergic; seasonal or perennial. Rhinitis may simply be related to whatever irritant is present in the child's environment, such as environmental tobacco smoke, or whatever virus is prevalent in the community. The symptoms of both sinusitis and upper respiratory tract infections, which overlap with those of rhinitis, will have similar, albeit more temporary, effects on sleep. The symptoms of rhinitis include nasal congestion, rhinorrhea, sneezing and—in the case of allergic rhinitis and even some viral upper respiratory tract infections—pruritis of the eyes, nose, and throat. Posterior nasal drainage can be exacerbated when the child is recumbent, particularly when first laying down to sleep, leading to difficulty with sleep onset as the child lays in bed sniffing, throat-clearing, and coughing.

Sleep-related symptoms associated with rhinitis include prolonged sleep onset latency, snoring, and sleep-disordered breathing ranging from increased upper airway resistance to overt obstructive sleep apnea syndrome. These sleep-related symptoms are primarily related to nasal congestion and inflammation. The importance of treating the sleep-related symptoms of rhinitis cannot be

Chidekel AS, ed. *Curbside Consultation in Pediatric Sleep Disorders: 49 Clinical Questions* (pp. 183-186)

Table 40-1

Respiratory Symptoms That May Cause Sleep Disruption

• Nasal congestion • Nasal pruritis • Cough	• Wheeze • Dyspnea • Chest pain or tightness

understated, as their consequences include daytime symptoms of sleepiness, decreased energy, and reduced quality of life. The treatment of rhinitis (primarily allergic rhinitis) targeting the major sleep disruptive symptom, nasal congestion, begins with intranasal corticosteroids. Nonsedating antihistamines and leukotriene receptor antagonists are also effective, although somewhat less so at addressing nasal congestion. Oral decongestants may cause insomnia and topical decongestants can improve nasal congestion acutely, but are not recommended for long-term use because of the risk of rhinitis medicamentosa, or rebound nasal congestion. Similarly, the sedating anti-histamines are also not recommended for long-term use because of their unfavorable side effect profile.

Asthma is another example of a chronic pediatric condition that can adversely impact sleep. With an incidence of approximately 10%, asthma is also a condition with which pediatric practitioners are highly familiar. Nocturnal asthma describes the presence of asthma symptoms—namely, cough, wheeze, and shortness of breath during nighttime sleeping hours. Nocturnal asthma is often a component of persistent asthma with symptoms that occur throughout the 24-hour cycle, but some children have asthma symptoms that predominate during the night. In fact, current asthma guidelines specifically recommend assessing nighttime asthma symptoms and sleep disruption as a part of routine asthma follow-up care. The assessment and treatment of nocturnal asthma begins with a standardized, guideline-driven approach and careful attention to the factors that may aggravate nocturnal asthma symptoms. In any patient with asthma, prescription of, and adherence to, the appropriate level of controller medication should be ensured. The child's sleep environment should be assessed for potential asthma triggers, such as dust mites, mold, or other irritants. Medical comorbidities, such as rhinitis or gastroesophageal reflux, should be evaluated and treated. It should also be noted that obstructive sleep apnea syndrome and snoring are known asthma comorbidities and may need to be assessed as well.

In both asthma and rhinitis, as well as in numerous other pediatric conditions, the presence of cough may create significant sleep problems. In general, rhinitis will cause a cough in the first half of the night, whereas asthma will cause increased coughing in the second half of the night. Suppurative lung diseases will cause coughing throughout the night. As such, cough can create problems with sleep onset, as well as contribute to significant sleep disruption and night wakings throughout the sleep period, resulting in significant impact on the daytime functioning of the child. However, the differential diagnosis of cough is quite broad, and a chronic cough, nocturnal or diurnal, will often require further evaluation to elucidate its true nature and provide treatment to resolution.

Acute or chronic pain from any cause will have a major impact on sleep (Table 40-2). Whether it is acute pain from surgery or an injury, or chronic pain from headaches, juvenile arthritis, or even fibromyalgia, the impact of pain on children's sleep and daytime function can be significant. Pain is associated with sleep onset and sleep maintenance insomnia, light and disrupted sleep, and increased wake time after sleep onset. Treatment of pain is critical to promote improved sleep

Table 40-2
Effects of Pain on Sleep

- Prolonged sleep latency
- Sleep disruption
- Increased wake time after sleep onset
- Decreased deep sleep (N3)
- Decreased REM sleep

quality and quantity, but pain medication—particularly narcotic pain medications—can worsen or unmask sleep-disordered breathing, causing both central and obstructive apnea, and decreasing drive to breathe, which increases the risk of hypoxia and hypercapnia.

Ensuring adequate and restorative sleep is a challenge in the face of any chronic condition or troublesome symptoms. Additional examples that the practitioner should consider include the sleep-disruptive effects of pruritis associated with eczema, as well as the pain, discomfort, and regurgitation that can be seen with gastroesophageal reflux. Gastroesophageal reflux may be particularly notable since the recumbent position may even promote esophageal reflux if not frank regurgitation. Finally, the symptoms of gastroesophageal reflux may be subtle, consisting of fussiness and sleep disruption in a young child, or dramatic if choking and coughing result in a sudden and frightening awakening.

Although they are often overlooked, caregivers of youth with acute and chronic medical conditions frequently experience significant disruptions to their sleep. As much as 85% of parents of youth with chronic illnesses have reported sleep disturbances. For example, a caregiver often has to take care of his or her child's health needs during the night, such as soothing itching from eczema or addressing pain concerns. In addition, parents may feel that they need to monitor their children's health status—for example, checking blood glucose levels for children with diabetes. For those children who are dependent on technology, such as heart monitors, alarms may go off and, thus, cause night awakenings. Finally, overall stress and anxiety can lead to significant sleep difficulties. The difficulties in caregivers' sleep have implications for overall health as these disturbances result in fatigue, irritability, stressed marital relationships, and depressed mood—all factors that can have a direct impact on child adjustment and quality of life.

It is crucial for us as providers to consider the impact of illness on sleep of the entire family. For those working with hospitalized youth, consider spreading out the checking of vitals when possible, so as to minimize middle of the night awakenings. In addition, whether in the hospital or at home, special care should be taken to maintain a quiet and dark sleep environment. Take care to dose pain medications so that their effectiveness peaks during night hours. In addition, always be cognizant of the impact that child illness may have on caregiver sleep and help the caregiver problem solve ways to minimize sleep disruption. Parents should be encouraged to maintain consistent sleep hygiene and habits after a diagnosis. For example, if your patient was sleeping independently prior to diagnoses, encourage the caregivers to maintain that routine and to enforce developmentally appropriate limit-setting at bedtime. By assessing sleep in both patients and caregivers at every clinic appointment, you can provide anticipatory guidance regarding the potential impact of illness on sleep and can help prevent these difficulties from escalating.

Suggested Readings

Link, H. What is nocturnal asthma? In: Chidekel, AS, ed. *Curbside Consultation in Pediatric Asthma: 49 Clinical Questions*. Thorofare, NJ: SLACK Incorporated; 2012:125-129.

Melzter, LJ, Davis, KF, Mindell, JA. Patient and parent sleep in a children's hospital. *Pediatric Nursing*. 2012;38,64-71.

Melzter, LJ, Moore, M. Sleep disruption in parents of children and adolescents with chronic illnesses: prevalence, causes, and consequences. *J Pediat Psychol*, 2008;33:279-292.

Palermo, TM, Owens, J. Introduction to the special issue: sleep in pediatric medical populations. *J Pediatr Psychol*. 2008;33:227-231.

Thompson, A, Sardana, N, Craig, TJ. Sleep impairment and daytime sleepiness in patients with allergic rhinitis: the role of congestion and inflammation. *Annals of Allergy Asthma and Immunology*. 2013;111,446-451.

QUESTION 41

What Are the Effects of Neuropsychiatric Disorders on Sleep?

Aaron S. Chidekel, MD

Many, if not all, of the more common (and uncommon) pediatric neuropsychiatric disorders can have a major impact on sleep (Table 41-1). While insomnia is generally the most common sleep-related comorbidity, changes in total sleep time, sleep latency, sleep architecture, and arousals and sleep disruption are commonly seen as well (Table 41-2). Coexistent sleep disorders, such as obstructive sleep apnea syndrome (OSAS) or periodic limb movement disorder, can occur as well and worsen sleep and daytime function. Treatments, particularly medical therapies for underlying insomnia, are poorly studied and anecdotal and there is even less experience with behavioral and other adjunctive therapies. Some pharmacological therapies for psychiatric conditions—such as anxiety, depression, and psychosis—have important effects on sleep in themselves and clinicians should be aware of these additional variables. Melatonin and clonidine are commonly used medical therapies for treating insomnia associated with conditions such as attention deficit hyperactivity disorder (ADHD) and autism/pervasive developmental disorder. Treating sleep problems in children with neuropsychiatric conditions is an ongoing challenge and remains a major unmet need for this important group of conditions.[1]

Attention Deficit Hyperactivity Disorder

Sleep problems are common among children with ADHD, in whom sleep-related complaints are present in as many as half of all children with this common pediatric condition.[2] Sleep-onset and maintenance insomnia are commonly reported, as children with ADHD may have difficulty settling or "turning off" at night. Further, children with ADHD are often described as light and restless sleepers. Polysomnographic findings in children with ADHD have included delayed sleep onset, sleep fragmentation, and reduced rapid eye movement (REM) time. To complicate matters, many of the symptoms of ADHD—namely inattention, impulsivity, and learning challenges—are

Chidekel AS, ed. *Curbside Consultation in Pediatric Sleep Disorders: 49 Clinical Questions* (pp. 187-190)

Table 41-1

Major Pediatric Neuropsychiatric Conditions Associated With Insomnia

• Autism • ADHD • Bipolar disorder • Generalized anxiety disorder	• Major depressive disorder • Mood disorder • Posttraumatic stress disorder • Separation anxiety disorder

Table 41-2

Common Polysomnographic Features of Pediatric Neuropsychiatric Conditions

- Increased sleep latency
- Increased wake time after sleep onset
- Increased arousals (sleep fragmentation)
- Decreased REM sleep
- Decreased non-REM Stage 3 sleep (deep sleep)
- Decreased total sleep time

also symptoms of sleep disorders and there is clearly overlap between ADHD and pediatric OSAS. Indeed, some children with ADHD actually have concurrent OSAS, which requires diagnosis and treatment. Inattentiveness and cognitive function and have been shown to improve after adenotonsillectomy—both in children with and without ADHD.[3,4] Careful screening for sleep-disordered breathing and sleep-related movements that may suggest periodic limb movements is particularly important when considering the diagnosis of ADHD and it is clear that some of these children will need further sleep evaluation as part of their diagnostic work-up. Treatment of ADHD with stimulant medications can compound sleep problems in this group of children. Attention to the timing, duration of action, and dosing of stimulant medications, therefore, is also critically important. Occasionally it will be necessary to attempt medical therapy of sleep-onset insomnia in children with ADHD, and melatonin and clonidine have been used for this purpose.

Autism/Pervasive Developmental Disorder

Autism encompasses a broad group of developmental and communication disorders, for which there is no known cause or cure. As in ADHD, sleep problems are common in autism (up to 50%

of children, if not more) and can be a tremendous challenge for children with this condition.[2] Polysomnographic features include light and disrupted sleep along with reduced sleep duration that is possibly biologically mediated. These culminate in both sleep onset and maintenance insomnia that can be severe and that can then feed back and contribute further to decrements in daytime functioning. Children with autism can experience prolonged night awakenings and their difficulty with social cues can result in inappropriate, disruptive, or noisy behaviors that result in the need for enhanced supervision that can quickly exhaust a family. Because of their underlying sensory and communication problems, children with autism can be particularly difficult to study in the sleep laboratory, where cooperation with a complex array of wires, sensors, and electrodes, which must be placed by a stranger in an unfamiliar setting to the child, is necessary. This has further limited the ability to collect data about sleep and autism. As in ADHD, evaluation for a comorbid, separate sleep disorder is as important since snoring, periodic limb movements, and other clinically relevant symptoms can occur and further worsen the child's sleep. As in ADHD, medical therapy for insomnia in autism has focused on the use of melatonin and clonidine, and one recent study highlighted a potential role for iron therapy in children with autism and restless sleep.[5] Despite this, a general lack of medical evidence makes treating sleep problems in autism a further challenge. Behavioral therapies are challenging in children with autism and, in the end, some parents resort to adjunctive therapies, such as weighted blankets and white noise machines, along with complementary and alternative medicine (CAM), to try and promote soothing, self-comfort, and sleep maintenance for their child.[6]

Anxiety and Depression

Separation anxiety and bedtime fears are common in all children during late toddlerhood and early school age. These types of issues, when they result in bedtime struggles or refusal, are often easily alleviated with supportive reassurance, a night light, and other common parenting strategies.[7] Generalized anxiety disorder is much more pervasive in the life of a child. It is a chronic disorder that is associated with a more complex and comprehensive array of symptoms. Sleep is impacted by generalized anxiety disorder, and sleep onset and maintenance insomnia is a common feature of this condition. Polysomnographically, sleep onset is delayed, sleep is light and disrupted, and wake time after sleep onset increases. In fact, there is a high incidence of current and lifetime insomnia in children and adolescents with generalized anxiety disorder. Posttraumatic stress disorder is also associated with similar sleep problems, with nightmares being an additional common feature. Treatment of the underlying anxiety disorder with medications and behavioral therapy can alleviate the sleep-related symptoms.

Major depressive disorder also has a high incidence of associated sleep-related problems, with as many as 75% of patients reporting sleep difficulties. Insomnia is common in major depressive disorder, and hypersomnia is reported as well. The evaluation and monitoring of sleep in patients with depression is further complicated by the role of medications, which is complex. There are many different types of antidepressant medications, which can have various effects on sleep and its architecture, and treating depression itself can also impact sleep concurrently. Most of the other psychiatric disorders, from bipolar disorder to the psychoses, all have major effects on sleep as well, but a detailed discussion of these is beyond the scope of this brief overview.

References

1. Mindell JA, Emslie G, Blumer J, et al. Pharmacologic management of insomnia in children and adolescents: consensus statement. *Pediatrics*. 2006;117(6):e1223-e1232.
2. Meltzer LJ, Mindel JA. Sleep and sleep disorders in children and adolescents. *Psychiatr Clin N Am*. 2006;29: 1059-1076.
3. Chervin RD, Archbold KH, Dillon JE, et al. Inattention, hyperactivity, and symptoms of sleep-disordered breathing. *Pediatrics*. 2002;109(3):449-456.
4. Chervin RD, Ruzicka DL, Giordani, BJ, et al. Sleep-disordered breathing, behavior and cognition in children before and after adenotonsillectomy. *Pediatrics*. 2006;117(4):e768-e769.
5. Dosman CF, Brian JA, Drmic IE, et al. Children with autism: effect of iron supplementation on sleep and ferritin. *Pediatr Neurol*. 2007;36(3):152-158.
6. Levy SE and Hyman SL. Complementary and alternative medicine treatments for children with autism spectrum disorders. *Child Adolesc Psychiatric Clin N Am*. 2008;17:803-820.
7. Hoban TF. Sleep and its disorders in children. *Semin Neurol*. 2004;24(3):327-340.

QUESTION 42

What Are the Effects of Medications on Sleep?

Aaron S. Chidekel, MD

Any medication that crosses the blood-brain barrier can have significant effects on sleep and arousal. These effects may be beneficial if a medication has the desired, or even therapeutic, effect on the sleep-wake cycle. The effect may be deleterious if the medication causes insomnia or drowsiness at an inopportune time. In addition to potential effects on the timing of wakefulness or sleep, medications can impact sleep architecture as measured during polysomnography (PSG). Common examples of this would include classes of medications, such as antidepressant agents, which suppress rapid eye movement (REM) sleep, and benzodiazepines, which suppress slow wave sleep. Additional effects of medications on sleep include causing or worsening periodic limb movements—also a potential effect of antidepressants—and causing or worsening parasomnias. Worsened parasomnias, and even bizarre sleep-related behaviors, have been reported with non-benzodiazepine gamma-amino butyric acid-A (GABA-A) agonists such as zolpidem, zaleplon, and eszopiclone. These medications are not approved by the United States Food and Drug Administration for use in children. These potentially powerful effects on sleep are not limited to prescription-only medications. Many over-the-counter medications, including those marketed as sleep aids, have important effects on the sleep-wake cycle as well. Finally, caffeine, a commonly used stimulant, is frequently used by adolescents seeking to maintain alertness in the face of an ever-increasing sleep debt.

Sleep is regulated behaviorally and biochemically. Medications will affect sleep by acting on central nervous system (CNS) sleep- and wake-promoting biochemical pathways (Table 42-1). A basic understanding of these pathways is useful in understanding how specific medications can impact sleep. In the CNS, arousal is mediated via the function of important neurotransmitters, such as acetylcholine, dopamine, histamine, norepinephrine, and serotonin. Sleep is promoted by the function of GABA and adenosine. Melatonin is an additional circadian-related sleep-promoting factor that will be discussed in Question 44. Medications that impact these pathways will either promote or inhibit sleep accordingly, and some examples of these relationships are shown in Table 42-2. The mechanism of action of the medication may be specifically targeted to this pathway, such as in the sleep-promoting effects of benzodiazepines via the GABA-ergic system. Conversely, the effect of a medication on sleep may be a side effect as is seen in the drowsiness

Chidekel AS, ed. *Curbside Consultation in Pediatric Sleep Disorders: 49 Clinical Questions* (pp. 191-194)

Table 42-1

Sleep-Mediating Neurotransmitter Systems

Wake-Promoting	
• Acetylcholine • Dopamine • Glutamate	• Histamine • Hypocretin/Orexin • Norepinephrine • Serotonin
Sleep-Promoting	
• Adenosine • GABA	

Table 42-2

Examples of Clinical/Pharmacological Interactions With Sleep-Mediating Neurotransmitters

Neurotransmitter System	*Clinical/Pharmacological Correlation*
Acetylcholine	Anticholinergic medications cause drowsiness
Histamine	First-generation antihistamines cause drowsiness
Hypocretin/Orexin	Deficiency in narcolepsy causes sleepiness
Norepinephrine	Stimulant medications cause insomnia
Adenosine	Adenosine antagonism by caffeine promotes wakefulness/insomnia

associated with the first-generation antihistamine medications. In the case of these first-generation antihistamines, this side effect allows these medications to be employed at times as sleep aids, albeit with limited efficacy. Interestingly, some of the other medications that are used off-label to treat pediatric sleep onset insomnia also make use of the side effect of drowsiness to promote sleep. For example, clonidine is an antihypertensive medication that causes drowsiness often used off-label to treat pediatric insomnia. The duration of action of a medication is important to consider as well as its specific mechanism of action. A medication that is sleep-promoting, but long-acting, may have continued effects, even after the main sleep period has ended, of residual sleepiness or morning fogginess. Although a complete discussion of all of the classes of medications and their possible effects on sleep is beyond the scope of this chapter, it is worth exploring some of the commonly prescribed classes of pediatric medications and understanding their potential effects on sleep.

Antidepressant medications have diverse effects on sleep, depending on the class of agent that is being prescribed. Older agents, such as tricyclic antidepressants, are generally sedating because of their anticholinergic and antihistaminic effects. Newer antidepressant medications tend to have the opposite effect. Selective serotonin reuptake inhibitors tend to be stimulating and can promote insomnia, decrease REM sleep, and increase periodic limb movements. Selective serotonin and norepinephrine reuptake inhibitors have similar effects on sleep. Examples of other antidepressants that may be sleep-promoting include trazodone and mirtazapine, which have diverse CNS effects (eg, antihistaminic effects and serotonin blockade). It should be apparent that, when prescribing these medications, a familiarity with their various and protean effects on sleep is critical. Other psychoactive medications of note include the antipsychotic medications, which are all generally sedating by a variety of mechanisms, and anxiolytic medications, such as benzodiazepines, which are also sedating. Similar to antidepressant medications, anticonvulsant medications can have variable effects on sleep. Some anticonvulsants, such as lamotrigine, can cause insomnia, while others, such as gabapentin, phenobarbital, and valproic acid are generally sedating.

Various classes of medications are more reliably known to cause insomnia. Stimulant medications used for the treatment of attention deficit hyperactivity disorder are, by their very nature, wake-promoting. Careful attention to the duration of action of these medications is important so as to minimally disrupt nighttime sleep onset. Similarly, anti-asthma medications tend to be arousing as well. Such medications as beta$_2$-agonists, theophylline (which is rarely used), and particularly systemic corticosteroids can all promote insomnia. Decongestants, such as pseudoephedrine and phenylpropanolamine, should also be used sparingly if at all in children, but can also cause significant insomnia as well.

Caffeine is a stimulant that requires special mention. Caffeine use is very common, particularly among adolescents, and its negative effects on sleep are well known and characterized. Caffeine is a centrally acting stimulant that acts directly on the CNS as an adenosine antagonist to promote arousal and inhibit sleep. Caffeine can prolong sleep onset latency even hours after being ingested. Caffeine is a common ingredient in coffee, soda, and energy drinks and it is ubiquitous in today's 24-hour society. It has important sleep-disrupting effects, particularly if ingested in the afternoon or early evening, which is when many adolescents drink caffeine. Asking directly about the ingestion of caffeine, its timing, and amount is critical when taking a sleep history, particularly among adolescents with sleep onset difficulties or even delayed sleep phase syndrome. Avoiding caffeine altogether, or at least eliminating caffeine intake after lunch, is an important component of good sleep hygiene.

Summary

The effects of medications on sleep are as diverse and broad as there are classes of medications. Furthermore, individual responses to medications may vary as well. Understanding the main wake- and sleep-promoting systems in the CNS can alert the practitioners to those medications that may be particularly important as they pertain to sleep-related effects. When prescribing a course of treatment, or a chronic medication, being aware of potential sleep-related effects is important. Similarly, when evaluating a patient with sleep difficulty or excessive sleepiness obtaining a full list of medications, prescription or otherwise, supplements and even drugs of abuse that a patient may be using is critical. Understanding the timing of the use of medications or supplements, particularly caffeine, and providing education to patients about the appropriate timing of their use will be beneficial as well. Finally, as part of the evaluation of a patient with a sleep disorder, it may even be necessary to obtain a toxicology screen.

Suggested Readings

Calamaro CJ, Mason TB, Ratcliffe SJ. Adolescents living the 24/7 lifestyle: effects of caffeine and technology on sleep duration and daytime functioning. *Pediatrics.* 2009;123:e1005-e1010.

Drake C, Roehrs T, shambroom J, Roth T. Caffeine effects on sleep taken 0, 3, or 6 hours before going to bed. *J Clin Sleep Med.* 2013;9(11):1195-1200.

Kothare SV, Kaleyias J. Sleep and epilepsy in children and adolescents. *Sleep Med.* 2010;11(7):674-685.

Merenstein D, Diener-West M, Halbower AC, Krist A, Rubin, HR. The trial of infant response to diphenhydramine: the TIRED study—a randomized, controlled, patient-oriented trial. *Arch Pediatr Adolesc Med.* 2006;160(7):707-712.

Pelayo R, Dubik M. Pediatric sleep pharmacology. *Semin Pediatr Neurol.* 2008;15(2):79-90.

QUESTION 43

Are There Any Medical Treatments for Insomnia in Children and Adolescents?

Aaron S. Chidekel, MD

It is normal for anyone to experience an occasional sleepless night, either due to difficulty falling to sleep or because of a prolonged nighttime awakening. Insomnia is more than an occasional sleepless night. True insomnia is characterized by persistent and repeated difficulty with the initiation or maintenance of sleep that occurs despite the provision of adequate opportunity and time for sleep and, critically, which results in daytime functional impairment. Many definitions of insomnia further characterize sleep difficulties as involving the duration and consolidation of sleep, as well as the concept that sleep is of insufficient quality to meet the needs of the individual. Finally, a pediatric definition of insomnia includes descriptors that allow for age-appropriateness and also recognizes the impact of a child's sleep difficulties or insomnia on the functioning of the family unit as well.[1] Recognizing the need for persistence of the symptoms and a quantifiable impact on daytime function or family dynamics is critical in differentiating true insomnia from occasional sleep difficulties or circadian rhythm sleep disorders.

In addition to the many other sleep-related challenges faced by adolescents, insomnia is actually quite common. Depending on the individual survey or definition for insomnia that is used in large cohort studies, reported lifetime prevalence rates for insomnia range from ~11%[2] to as high as nearly 24%.[3] Insomnia is consistently reported more frequently in females than males, and many of the adolescents surveyed in these studies reported current insomnia.[2] Children and adolescents with neurodevelopmental, psychiatric, and medical comorbidities have an even greater propensity to experience chronic insomnia (Table 43-1). Pediatric practitioners should be particularly aware of the potential for insomnia in children with neurological and psychiatric conditions, such as pervasive developmental disorders, attention deficit hyperactivity disorder, mood and anxiety disorder, as well as such diagnoses as asthma, cancer, and chronic pain.

The diagnosis of insomnia is made with a thorough clinical and sleep history supported by physical examination. Important questions are listed in Table 43-2. It is often useful to try to differentiate difficulties with sleep onset from sleep maintenance problems and further explore

Chidekel AS, ed. *Curbside Consultation in Pediatric Sleep Disorders: 49 Clinical Questions* (pp. 195-199)

Table 43-1

Selected Conditions Associated With Pediatric and Adolescent Insomnia

Neurodevelopmental Conditions
• Pervasive developmental disorders • Autism • Asperger's syndrome • Attention deficit hyperactivity disorder • Developmental disabilities • Tic disorders
Psychiatric Conditions
• Anxiety disorder • Bipolar disorder • Depression • Substance abuse
Medical Conditions
• Asthma • Cancer • Cerebral palsy • Childhood epilepsy syndromes • Chronic pain syndromes • Cystic fibrosis • Rheumatologic disorders

whether sleep is restful and restorative. Finally, it is also important to assess the teenager's level of distress or concern about their sleep as well. In order to meet criteria for insomnia, one or more nighttime symptoms must be present for 4 or more times per week for at least 1 month or more, and a patient must also exhibit daytime concern or distress about their sleep. A frank and detailed discussion of sleep hygiene is important and often provides insight into areas where interventions can be started. Finally, direct questioning about medications, caffeine, or other substance use is important as well. Distinguishing insomnia from a circadian rhythm sleep disorder, such as delayed sleep phase syndrome (DSPS), is not difficult since, unlike those with insomnia, individuals with DSPS have normal sleep latency, normal sleep quality and quantity, and awaken refreshed when allowed to sleep according to their preferred schedule. Asking about weekends, vacations, and sleeping at hotels or friends' houses can help to tease these issues out. Polysomnography is not usually indicated or necessary to make the diagnosis of insomnia unless other symptoms of a respiratory or nonrespiratory sleep disorder are present.

At the present time, there is a strong need for further studies of both the pharmacological and nonpharmacological management of pediatric/adolescent insomnia.[1] Nonpharmacological strategies are often inferred from the adult literature, and pharmacological strategies are both

Table 43-2

Assessment of Insomnia

Sleep Initiation • Do you have trouble falling asleep when you want to? • Does it take you an hour or longer to fall asleep after going to bed?
Sleep Maintenance • Do you awaken often at night after falling to sleep? • When you awaken at night is it difficult for you to return to sleep?
Nonrestorative Sleep • Do you awaken refreshed and ready for the day after sleeping? • Do you ever feel fatigued during the day due to poor sleep quality?
Concern About Sleep • Do you worry about having trouble sleeping? • Are you sad or frustrated about your trouble sleeping? • Does your trouble sleeping make it hard for you to do the things you usually do?

off-label and based on limited evidence. Nonpharmacological therapies for adult insomnia include behavioral techniques—such as sleep restriction, stimulus control, and cognitive therapy—about which there are limited data in children and adolescents. Similarly, there have been a few studies evaluating pharmacological options, such as melatonin, zolpidem, and clonidine, mostly in children and adolescents with underlying neurobehavioral conditions such as attention deficit/hyperactivity disorder.[4,5] In general, this scant literature has demonstrated a mild improvement in sleep-related symptoms with both clonidine and melatonin. Clonidine generally improved sleep parameters, whereas melatonin specifically improved sleep-onset latency, sleep efficiency, and total sleep time in some studies and conditions. Zolpidem, which is not approved by the Food and Drug Administration (FDA) for use in children under the age of 18 years, was not efficacious and resulted in side effects. The reader is specifically referred to Barrett, Tracy, and Giaroli[4] for a review of this literature. A number of other classes of medications with sedative or hypnotic properties (or side effects) have been used to treat pediatric and adolescent insomnia, as noted in Table 43-3, but the use of these medications for this purpose is neither well-studied nor evidence-based.[4-6]

Behavioral therapy of adolescent insomnia is multifaceted and requires a careful evaluation of all of the factors that may be contributing to poor sleep in an adolescent.[7] These factors are protean and need to be discussed frankly if progress is to be made. Biological factors, including an inherent circadian phase delay, favor a later bedtime, whereas societal factors, such as early school start times, and multiple and competing social demands serve to limit the opportunity for an adolescent to sleep as well. Examples of other factors that influence sleep hygiene and increase the risk of insomnia, as well as DSPS and simple sleep restriction, include an

Table 43-3

Medications Used Off-Label as Sleep-Aids in Pediatric/ Adolescent Patients Listed Alphabetically

- Alpha-adrenergic agonists
- Antidepressant medications
- Antiepileptic medications
- Antihistamine medications (sedating)
- Antipsychotic medications
- Barbiturate medications
- Benzodiazepine medications
- Herbal remedies
- Hypnotic medications
- Melatonin
- Over-the-counter sleep medications

Adapted from Barrett JR, Tracy DK, Giaroli G. To sleep or not to sleep: a systematic review of the literature of pharmacological treatments of insomnia in children and adolescents with attention-deficit/ hyperactivity disorder. *J Child Adolesc Psychopharmacol* 2013;23(10):640-647; and Phillips L, Appleton RE. Systematic review of melatonin treatment in children with neurodevelopmental disabilities and sleep impairment. *Dev Med Child Neurol.* 2004;46(11):771-775.

unfavorable sleep environment (electronics in the bedroom), the lack of parentally enforced bedtime, and the poorly timed use of stimulants, such as caffeine. School sports or other activities that last into the evening and academic demands are further stressors on the sleep of an adolescent. Evaluating and managing these factors requires specific questioning to delineate them and buy-in from the teenager and his or her parents in order to be impactful. Helpful concepts include stressing the importance of a consistent bedtime and wake time, the limitation of daytime naps, the avoidance of caffeine and other stimulants, and promoting a cool, dark and electronics-free bedroom environment that is conducive to sleep onset and maintenance.

Summary

The diagnosis of insomnia in adolescence is common and multifactorial. Intrinsic biological changes associated with adolescent sleep, along with the complex interplay of social and societal demands, contribute to the risk of insomnia and other adolescent sleep problems. Insomnia is diagnosed based on specific criteria, polysomnography is rarely indicated, and treatment is not particularly evidence-based. Pharmacological therapy is off-label and poorly studied, and behavioral therapy is complex and multifaceted. Behavioral therapy is based on principles of sound sleep hygiene and parental involvement.

References

1. Mindell JA, Emslie G, Blumer J, et al. Pharmacologic management of insomnia in children and adolescents: Consensus Statement. *Pediatrics*. 2006;117(6):e1223-e1232.
2. Johnson EO, Roth T, Schultz L, Breslau N. Epidemiology of DSM-IV insomnia in adolescence: lifetime prevalence, chronicity, and an emergent gender difference. *Pediatrics* 2006;117(2):e247-e256.
3. Hysing M, Pallesen S, Stormark KM, et al. Sleep patterns and insomnia among adolescents: a population-based study. *J Sleep Res*. 2013; 22:549-556.
4. Barrett JR, Tracy DK, Giaroli G. To sleep or not to sleep: a systematic review of the literature of pharmacological treatments of insomnia in children and adolescents with attention-deficit/hyperactivity disorder. *J Child Adolesc Psychopharmacol*. 2013;23(10):640-647.
5. Phillips L, Appleton RE. Systematic review of melatonin treatment in children with neurodevelopmental disabilities and sleep impairment. *Dev Med Child Neurol*. 2004;46(11):771-775.
6. Owens JA, Rosen CL, Mindell JA: Medication use in the treatment of pediatric insomnia: results of a survey of community-based pediatricians. *Pediatrics*. 2003;111(5):e628-e635.
7. Carskadon MA. Sleep in adolescents: the perfect storm. *Pediatr Clin N Am*. 2011;58:637-647.

44 QUESTION

What Is Melatonin and Is This an Effective Treatment for Insomnia?

Aaron S. Chidekel, MD

Melatonin Physiology

Melatonin is a hormone that is synthesized and secreted by the pineal gland from its main precursors—tryptophan and serotonin. Its synthesis and secretion maintains a tight circadian rhythm that is timed with the onset of ambient darkness or night and, therefore, melatonin secretion should ideally be timed to correspond with the arrival of the main sleep period or, in pediatric parlance, bedtime! As such, melatonin can be considered to be the primary circadian signal of night and sleep, whereas ambient light is considered to be the primary circadian signal of day and wakefulness. As part of a well-synchronized biological clock and circadian rhythm, melatonin secretion should commence in the evening with the fall off of ambient light and signal the onset of biological night to the rest of the body. Ambient light stimulation in the evening can delay the onset of melatonin secretion and biological nightfall and, therefore, bedtime. Conversely, exposure to early morning light can decrease melatonin secretion and promote wakefulness. Melatonin secretion should remain high during the main sleep period and its secretion should begin to fall off toward the arrival of biological and circadian day to promote wakefulness. Studies of the secretion of melatonin in humans clearly show this rhythmicity with melatonin secretion commencing with the onset of darkness, peaking in the middle of the sleep period in the wee hours of the morning, and then falling off thereafter toward daybreak and the light of the dawn.

With its tight circadian and light-dark regulation, melatonin synthesis and secretion is closely related to the function of the suprachiasmatic nucleus (SCN), which, as discussed in Question 3, is the major determinant of the human circadian rhythm. Indeed, the secretion of melatonin in response to ambient darkness is the main inhibitory signal to the SCN signaling that night has arrived. The central role of melatonin in the transduction of ambient darkness to biological night and sleep has lead to great interest in the use of melatonin in adult sleep disorders, such as shift-work sleep disorder and jetlag, which will not be discussed in this chapter. Rather, the potential role of exogenous melatonin in the treatment of sleep onset insomnia in children will be examined.

Chidekel AS, ed. *Curbside Consultation in Pediatric Sleep Disorders: 49 Clinical Questions* (pp. 201-203)

Melatonin as a Supplement

Currently, melatonin is only available in the United States as a dietary supplement and, as such, it is not available by prescription and it is not regulated by the Food and Drug Administration. It should only be taken in its synthetic form, rather than derived from bovine pineal gland, and families need to be aware that there may differences in co-ingredients, dosing consistency, bioavailability, and formulation, depending on the melatonin preparation that is purchased. Melatonin is available in various formulations (pills, liquids, chewable tablets) and various dosages of up to 10 mg. In addition, supplements of melatonin precursors (tryptophan, 5-hydroxytryptophan) are also available, but these are even less well studied than melatonin and are likely to be even less potent or effective than melatonin. At the pharmacological doses available for use as a supplement, it is likely that melatonin has a mild, intrinsic hypnotic effect, but the main role of melatonin in the body is as a circadian timing signal, rather than as a sedative or hypnotic per se. Melatonin, in any dose or formulation has, as its main role, the signaling to the SCN that night has arrived and that other rhythmic biological activities, such as body temperature, bowel, and bladder function, should be adjusted accordingly. Pediatric practitioners should also be aware that there is a melatonin receptor agonist medication (ramelteon) that is available and has been approved by the United States Food and Drug Administration for the treatment of adult sleep onset insomnia. This medication, which is sleep-promoting because of its stimulation of melatonin receptors in the brain, is not approved for use in children and is only mentioned here for the sake of completeness.

Brief Review of the Evidence

Studies of melatonin in the treatment of pediatric insomnia are extremely limited. In fact, this literature consists of a few brief and short-term studies in children with neurodevelopmental disabilities and attention deficit hyperactivity disorder, so it is quite difficult to objectively draw conclusions about the efficacy and safety of melatonin use in general pediatric practice and on outcomes, such as total sleep time, latency to falling asleep, and nighttime awakenings. In children with neurodevelopmental disabilities, such as developmental delays, autism, seizures, and visual impairment, it is likely that melatonin supplementation has a modest effect on sleep latency of approximately 20 to 30 minutes, but minimal, if any, impact on total sleep time or nighttime awakenings. Similarly, it is likely that melatonin has a similarly modest effect on sleep latency and total sleep time in children with ADHD and chronic sleep onset insomnia. Given this almost total lack of evidence regarding efficacy, it is similarly difficult to truly define the safety of melatonin treatment as well. In general, melatonin is thought to be safe for short-term use and there are no reports in the few published studies of significant adverse events or side effects and no case reports of adverse events are noted in the medical literature.

Potential Use of Melatonin in Clinical Practice

Because melatonin use in clinical practice cannot be strictly guided by medical evidence, it should be grounded in common sense and conservatism. The treatment of pediatric sleep onset insomnia should start with a clear emphasis on the principles of sleep hygiene and regularity and only after these behavioral and environmental factors have been addressed should additional pharmacological options such as melatonin be discussed. When implemented, melatonin should be used at the lowest efficacious dose, at a time that is logical given its role as a biological timing signal and in concert with the implementation of a bedtime ritual that will also serve to promote the onset of sleep. Ideally, melatonin should be given in a dimly lit and quiet setting, approximately 30 to 60 minutes prior to bedtime, and in a child who is growing sleepy anyway. Melatonin, therefore, should be given to complement the child's intrinsic homeostatic sleep drive, at the right time of day to signal the onset of biological night since it will not promote sleep as a sedative or hypnotic agent. Once the child has learned to fall asleep with a robust and consistently timed bedtime ritual and good sleep hygiene, consideration should be given to stopping the melatonin. Finally, it should be remembered that even the limited published data regarding melatonin shows little effect on nighttime awakenings and, therefore, the use of melatonin for sleep maintenance insomnia or struggles simply cannot be recommended.

Suggested Readings

Doghramji K. Melatonin and its receptors: a new class of sleep-promoting agents. *J Clin Sleep Med.* 2007; 3(5):S17-S23.

Arendt J, Rajaratnam SMW. Melatonin and its agonists: an update. *Br J Psychiatry.* 2008;193:267-269.

Phillips L, Appleton RE. Systematic review of melatonin treatment in children with neurodevelopmental disabilities and sleep impairment. *Dev Med Child Neurol.* 2004;46:771-775.

Bendz LM, Scates AC. Melatonin treatment for insomnia in pediatric patients with attention deficit/hyperactivity disorder. *Annals of Pharmacotherapy*: 2010;44(1):185-191.

Hoebert M, van der Heijden, van Geiglswijk, Smits MG. Long-term follow-up of melatonin treatment in children with ADHD and chronic sleep onset insomnia. *J Pineal Res.* 2009;47(1):1-7.

SECTION VIII

SLEEP EVALUATION AND TESTING

QUESTION 45

How Do I Screen for Sleep Problems in My Practice?

Lewis J. Kass, MD

Many children have trouble sleeping. Sleep problems can occur at all ages from birth through adolescence and, frequently, the pediatrician is on the front line. Sometimes the sleep issue comes up in the course of a routine well-child visit, and sometimes it is the parent who raises the concern. Parents can sometimes feel lost not knowing whether what they see in their child is a small problem or a big problem, or whether it is even a problem at all. This is where a pediatric sleep consultation comes in. The complete assessment should include an in-depth history and a comprehensive physical examination. This is then generally followed, if necessary, by an overnight sleep study.

When there are more than one child in a household, invariably a parent's reference point is another sibling. If the first child started sleeping through the night at 3 months of age and the second child is 8 months old and is still not sleeping through the night, a parent understandably cannot help but wonder if their second child is "normal." Parents frequently use phrases like "he's an awful sleeper" or "she's horrible at night" or "his sleep is killing us all" or "she's never been a good sleeper."

After first cringing when a parent says that in front of the child, I then try to break down a parent's concerns into some easily defined categories:

- Is it a concern about falling asleep?
- Is it about trouble staying asleep?

At that point I find it very helpful to have a parent take me through a child's 24-hour day, starting at bedtime. It is important to distinguish between bedtime, lights out, head on pillow, and sleep onset. They can all have similar meanings in a parent's mind, but mean vastly different things when trying to establish the meaning of sleep onset. For example, if you ask what time bedtime is, a parent might describe the beginning of the nighttime routine. They might respond: "6 p.m." Great, right? But what if 6 p.m. is when they start running a bath, followed by coaxing and cajoling to get into pajamas and brushing teeth? Now it's 7:30 and reading in bed starts—followed by kisses and goodnights. Now it is 8 p.m. and suddenly you realize that bedtime at 6 p.m. really means the time of starting the bedtime routine, and the actual bedtime and lights out is not until 8 p.m.

Chidekel AS, ed. *Curbside Consultation in Pediatric Sleep Disorders: 49 Clinical Questions* (pp. 207-210)

Once sleep time is established, I segue momentarily into sleep quality. Is the child restless or does he sleep like a rock? Does he snore? Does she sweat in her sleep? Does she kick her legs? Does he wet the bed? Bedwetting takes on particular significance in the sleep world because obstructive sleep apnea can be a source of or contributor to the bedwetting.

The topic of nocturnal enuresis can then bring you down a long pathway of questioning. Try not to get lost; remember we are still trying to understand first about a child's sleep and wake schedule. Is it primary or secondary enuresis? Does he wear a pull-up to sleep? Does he soak the pull-up? Parents will be very descriptive about surprisingly large volumes of urine. Have there been any other consultations about the bedwetting? Nephrology? Urology? Psychology? Have any interventions been attempted? Water regulation? Medication? Planned awakenings to void? Alarms? Hypnosis?

Returning to the schedule: Does he wake up? What time is that? How many times does he wake up? Does he call out for you? Do you respond? How do you respond? Does he climb into bed with you? Once in bed with you, is he restless or does he sleep like a rock? The time of the awakening or the behaviors and actions after the awakening might help point you in the direction of whether you are dealing with night terrors, sleepwalking, or even seizures.

What time is wake up for the day? Is it easy for her to wake up? Do you ever miss the bus because it is hard to get her up? Is she late for school? Does your child feel sleepy in school? Is her head nodding? Dozing? Does your child ever put her head down on the desk to sleep? If so, are there dreams? Are there any trips to the nurse's office to nap? While in school, are there issues with focus? concentration? impulsivity? hyperactivity? How are the school grades?

What time does your child come home? Is there energy for homework? Is there head nodding during homework? Any after school activities? Is there energy for those activities? What time do you come home from those activities? Is there any napping when you get home? What time is dinner? Is homework done before or after dinner? before or after after-school activities? All of these questions help define the true amount of sleepiness.

After dinner, how much time is spent on an electronic device (television, tablet, smart phone, computer, laptop, video game)? What time does the device go off for the night? These questions are aimed at understanding more about whether daily routine schedule is a problem and whether exposure to light-emitting electronic devices after sunset might be altering the intrinsic circadian rhythm and possibly delaying bedtime.

At some point, one should ask about any chronic pains or other medical problems, such as asthma, allergies, cough, headaches, leg discomfort, or prolonged cough with colds.

This then usually gets us back to bedtime. At some point in the history-taking process, it might become clear whether the sleep problem is behavioral or not. If a child is not restless during sleep or, once a child comes into bed with the parent he or she does not move at all, then this may point to behavioral issues.

From the history alone, a pretty good differential diagnosis can be generated. Between physical exam and sleep testing, all should become clear.

The physical exam for a sleep consultation starts during the history-taking. Is the child awake or asleep? yawning? hyperactive? impulsive? clingy? fearful? Can he be redirected and corralled? (ie, Is he a good listener? Is he moody? Does he have a short fuse? Does she have tantrums?)

Is the child obese? Is he underweight? Is breathing audible from across the room?

Does he bounce his legs rhythmically or repeatedly? If you point out the leg bouncing and ask him to try not bouncing them, is he able to do it? An inability to stop bouncing legs might point toward restless legs syndrome.

Does he have big tonsils or a hyponasal voice? These answers might point you toward obstructive sleep apnea. It should always be remembered, though, that having small tonsils does not rule out obstructive sleep apnea.

Is the oropharynx red, cobblestoned, or inflamed? These might be clues about acid reflux, post-nasal drip, or allergies.

The lung exam is important and is frequently overlooked in a sleep visit. Remember that breathing is the most primal drive that we possess. Our brains would sooner wake us up 100 times per hour than allow us to sleep and have trouble breathing. In babies with their small noses and small nasal passages and small airways, this is an especially important point. Asthma can be a potent sleep disturber and can sometimes only be considered after hearing surprisingly distant breath sounds. You may sometimes be fortunate enough to hear a wheeze. Auscultation can also point you in the direction of laryngotracheomalacia (collapsible vocal cords and/or trachea) as a source of trouble breathing. In a child who is old enough, such findings might prompt you to do pulmonary function testing before leaping to a costly overnight sleep study.

Vital signs are also important. Obstructive sleep apnea can elevate blood pressure or lead to a higher than expected resting heart rate or respiratory rate. Is there even wakeful hypoxemia seen by pulse oximetry? What is the body mass index?

The rest of the physical exam can also give you clues. Is there muscle weakness that might predispose to restrictive hypoventilation at night? Is a baby's belly distended with gas? Could this represent milk intolerance? Milk intolerance can predispose to acid reflux or belly pain—either of which can cause nighttime awakenings or difficulty falling asleep. If milk protein allergy leads to microscopic blood loss, then this can lead to limb movements and restless legs—another potent disturber of sleep. Is the skin blotchy and eczematous? This might then point to allergies; yet another disturber of sleep.

This then brings us to the in-lab overnight sleep study (polysomnography), which will confirm or refute your suspicions. It may identify a problem that was not even considered. It will provide an objective measure with which to make decisions and advocate for treatment. In an ideal world, it would be performed in a pediatric sleep center, by pediatric sleep technicians, and reviewed and interpreted by a board-certified pediatric sleep physician. Depending on geography, this may or may not be realistic, but aiming for the ideal gives you the best chance of taking the best possible care of your patients. Sleep centers that do not take care of many children may not be experienced enough to complete a study in a young, nervous, or combative child. Studies completed, but interpreted by an adult sleep physician, may be underscored and misinterpreted.

These days, the adult sleep world has been overtaken by the insurance and cost-driven practice of performing sleep studies at home (home sleep testing). Thus far in pediatrics, we have been immune to this, but no doubt the push is around the corner. We will need to push back. There has also been a revenue-driven force to have board-certified pediatric sleep doctors interpret studies remotely with the interpreting doctor never having seen the patient. This, too, is a bad practice and should be avoided. In order to make an accurate diagnosis, every aspect of care needs to be taken together—history, physical examination, and polysomnography.

All of the above explains my approach to a child with a possible sleep problem. It is certainly understandable that, in a busy pediatric practice, there may not be time to delve so deeply into all the facets of a sleep consultation. However, if I had just 3 or 4 questions that I could ask, they would be:

1. Is your child restless?
2. Does she sweat in her sleep?
3. Does she snore?
4. Does she wake up from sleep?

If the answer is yes to any or all of those questions, then a pediatric sleep consultation would probably be a pretty good idea.

Suggested Readings

Babcock DA. Evaluating sleep and sleep disorders in the pediatric primary care setting. *Pediatric Clinics of North America.* 2011;58(3):543-554.

Moore M, Allison D, Rosen CL. A review of pediatric nonrespiratory sleep disorders. *Chest.* 2006;130(4):1252-1262.

Owens JA, Dalzell V. Use of the 'BEARS' sleep screening tool in a pediatric residents' continuity clinic: a pilot study. *Sleep Med.* 2005;6(1):63-69.

46 QUESTION

How Can I Promote Sleep Hygiene in My Practice?

Jennifer A. Marriner, MSN, CPNP

Good sleep hygiene is the terminology we use to convey the idea that the routine and environment in which one sleeps should be ideal to promote sleep. Children and adolescents are particularly vulnerable to poor and inadequate amounts of sleep for many reasons, including a lack of insight regarding the short- and long-term consequences of insufficient sleep. Infants and young children need to learn how to settle and sleep through the night. It is up to those caring for children to establish and enforce good bedtime routines and instill good sleep habits to ensure that adequate sleep and sleep hygiene habits become life-long. It is important for us as health care providers to assess our patients' sleep and to educate their parents about the promotion and maintenance of quality sleep and to help parents and families promote good sleep hygiene for their children.

The promotion of good sleep hygiene should begin at birth. Infants are known to sleep a significant portion of most days (between 16 to 20 hours), with their sleep being fragmented and irregular and divided between the day and night due to not having a fully entrained internal clock. New and exhausted parents are often frustrated and do not know what to expect. Variability exists among newborns, so that not all infants sleep and act the same or according to parental expectations. Parents of newborns who sleep and eat well are considered fortunate. Temperament plays a role in how a baby soothes and sleeps as does the temperament of the parents and their ability to handle the stress of a new baby and sleep disruption that can accompany caring for a new baby. The establishment of a consistent routine to promote security and set expectations pays long-term dividends for parents. Placing an infant who is drowsy, but awake, down to sleep and encouraging him or her to drift off alone in early infancy is a way to combat full wakefulness later when the baby stirs.

Well-meaning parents wanting to do the right thing often rescue a distressed infant to aid and assist him or her. Crying is viewed negatively instead of as a natural and healthy response. Parents want to do something to stop the crying and the infant quickly learns to associate the parent as a condition for settling. Rocking, patting, walking, and feeding to soothe a baby to sleep negatively reinforces a sleep onset association that often becomes difficult to break later as the baby matures.

Chidekel AS, ed. *Curbside Consultation in Pediatric Sleep Disorders: 49 Clinical Questions* (pp. 211-213)

Beginning in the newborn period, all well-child visits should encompass how the baby is sleeping and how the family is doing with sleep. If parents hear how important sleep is for their child and how much you value it and their well being as the health care provider, they will note that it is a part of what will be asked of them at each visit and, therefore, it must be important. You should address sleeping much like feeding. Reviewing at each well visit what the usual requirements are for that child's developmental level, while stressing that all children are different, gives parents a general idea of how their baby is doing and what they might expect based on his or her developmental level. Parents do not always bring up sleep in the time crunch of a well visit unless they feel that it is an extreme problem or it has become distressing. Some parents also believe that some scenarios are normal or to be expected when they may well be unreasonable. Parents need to understand and believe that some refinements and consistent management early on can save time and eliminate undue stress later and are what is best for their child.

Parents should be provided with age-specific guidelines and information at each well visit (Table 46-1). You may do this easily with sleep printouts from your computer or you can have readily available handouts in the office. Information is easily and cheaply attainable. Handouts or information on a suitable sleep environment and bedtime routines, as well as common sleep-related issues in children (such as night waking, nightmares, fears, and head banging), may also be given. Parents can read these later at their convenience or refer to them as needed.

Sleep problems and complaints are estimated to occur in about 25% of children.[1] Disturbed and inadequate sleep in children is thought to be extensive and significant. The effects of poor and disturbed sleep are thought to have an impact on children's cognitive development, mood regulation, attention and behavior, as well as on their health and overall quality of life.[2] If parents understand this concept, they may choose to prioritize sleep. Health care providers need to emphasize and assess not only children's sleep quantity, but also the parents' belief that it is as important as nutrition and growth, learning, and play. For those with problems beyond the basics, a referral to a pediatric sleep specialist can help tease out medical and more significant behavioral problems.

Table 46-1

Clinical Pearls for Good Sleep Hygiene in Children of All Ages

Sleep Hygiene at All Ages

- A regular daily schedule
- Healthy sleep environment that is conducive to sleep
  - Cool, dark, and quiet
- Morning light exposure

Infant and Toddler Age

- Establish regular sleep schedule including regular scheduled naps
- Establish bedtime routine:
  - Bath, book, bed
- Transitional objects as developmentally appropriate
- Avoid falling asleep or sleeping in an environment other than own crib or bed
- Avoid bright lights in the bedroom during the night
- Avoid pitfall of nighttime feeding

School Age

- Maintain consistent routine
- Reduce stimulating play at bedtime
- Set regular bedtime and wake time
- No electronics in the bedroom
- Avoid caffeine intake
- Be aware of the challenge of evening sports and activities

Adolescence

- Set appropriate bedtime for 9 hours of sleep
- Get up at a reasonable time on weekends to avoid difficulty with sleep Sunday night
- Morning light exposure
- Limit electronics in the bedroom
- Eliminate caffeine intake after noon
- Be aware of the challenge of evening sports, jobs, and activities

References

1. Owens J. Classification and epidemiology of childhood sleep disorders. *Sleep Med Clin*. 2007;2(3):353-361.
2. Sadeh A. Consequences of sleep loss or sleep disruption in children. *Sleep Med Clin*. 2007;2(3):513-520.

QUESTION 47

What Is a Polysomnogram?

Todd Burchard, BS, RPSGT, RST and Aaron S. Chidekel, MD

In order to assure that the patient's overnight stay is as pleasant as possible, and to attach the needed devices to the patient as successfully as possible to obtain quality signals, strong effort should be made to create an environment in which the patient is relaxed and cooperative. A sleep center can do several things to help the patient be compliant with the sleep technologist's instructions and avoid a polysomnogram (PSG) with limited channels, or early termination of the study. A pediatric sleep center should have the necessary supplies and amenities to accommodate patients, of newborn age to early adulthood, as well as taking into consideration the needs of parents and guardians (eg, disposable toothbrushes) since a guardian is required to stay with the patient throughout the night. Children get their cues from parents, so creating comfort by explaining to both the child and guardian what to expect, how long the set up and study will take, and why the devices are being used, is crucial.

Parents/guardians are encouraged to bring a "comfort item" for the child, such as a blanket or stuffed bear, and the sleep laboratory should also have a supply of a range of age-appropriate books, toys, and other comfort items that can be easily cleaned. Children and parents can bring their own pillows, pajamas, and slippers. Parents should also be given clear instructions as to what the sleep center cannot provide. Many sleep centers do not provide medications or meals, and parents should be informed of that before coming for testing. Television and electronics are discouraged before bedtime, but, in many cases, they can be used as tools to distract the patient while the technologist applies the sensors. The technologist can enlist the parent to help apply items that the child does not feel comfortable having the technologist apply.

An experienced technologist is critical to a successful setup. For example, one successful method of placing electroencephalogram (EEG) electrodes is to start by showing the patient the electrodes first, then having the technician place the electrode on their own hand, then having the patient place the electrode on the technician's hand, or their parent's hand, then on their own hand. Be careful with using words such as *electrodes*. Patients often hear the word *electric* and are afraid they will be shocked. Calling electrodes *buttons* or *stickers* can help lessen the anxiety. Once

Chidekel AS, ed. *Curbside Consultation in Pediatric Sleep Disorders: 49 Clinical Questions* (pp. 215-220)

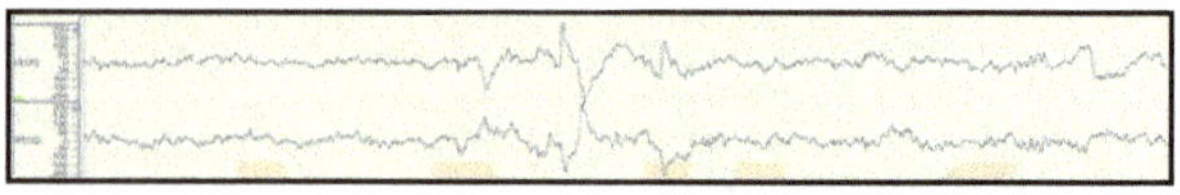

Figure 47-1. EOG channels depicting sharp eye movements.

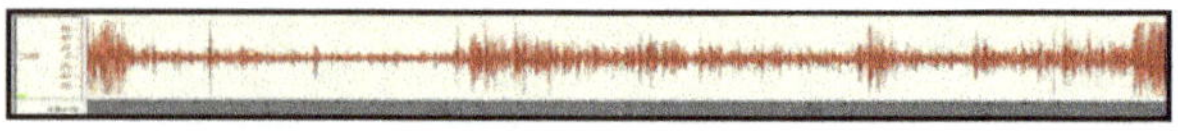

Figure 47-2. Chin EMG recording depicting chin muscle activity.

the EEGs are placed on the patient's head, often laboratories wrap the patient's head in gauze to help prevent the electrodes from coming off during the night.

Rewards also serve as a helpful tool. A technologist can offer stickers to accomplish patient compliance. In some cases, the technologist may not be able to place an item on the patient until after they fall asleep. In rare cases, the technologist may not be able to place some items on the patient at all. The patient's safety must be taken into account when determining whether or not to record a limited-channel PSG. Such channels as the SpO_2 or ECG channels must be monitored, and the patient's medical history must also be taken into account.

PSGs record multiple channels, for multiple reasons, but one of the primary reasons is to detect sleep and to identify the type of sleep. Sleep is broken into 2 parts: rapid eye movement (REM), and non-REM (NREM). NREM is further broken down to 3 parts: N1, N2, and N3. These parts are termed *stages*. Each PSG recording's sleep is staged in 30-second intervals or pages, called an epoch. Several pairs of electrodes, termed *channels*, are recorded to identify the sleep stages, most importantly the (EEG), along with the electrooculogram (EOG) used to detect eye movement, and the chin EMG used to detect chin atonia. Each epoch of these combined channels are reviewed by a technologist and staged according to American Academy of Sleep Medicine (AASM) standards.

The EEG signals, or channels, are recorded by using electrodes that are placed on the scalp in certain locations using the international 10-20 measurement system. The 10-20 system is a measurement and placement system developed to assure accuracy of scalp electrode placement, in regards to the cerebral cortex. The measurement system is based on frontal lobe (F), temporal lobe (T), central sulcus (C), parietal lobe (P), occipital lobe (O), and mastoid (M) locations, with the goal of a standard format, correct locations, and uniform terminology. Each 10-20 placement has an identifier, one letter, and one number (eg, C-3). The letter corresponds to the location of the brain, and the number further identifies its placement. Even numbers are used to indicate placement on the right side of the patient's brain, and odd to indicate placement on the left.

The EEG locations required by the AASM are F3, F4, C3, C4, O1, O2, and are referenced to the opposing mastoid locations M1 or M2 (formerly A1 and A2), resulting in the current standard PSG EEG montage: F3-M2, F4-M1, C3-M2, C4-M1, O1-M2, O2-M1. The rejection of unwanted material, along with high- and low-frequency filters that narrow in to the desired wave range, will result in the output of the sought-after EEG signal.

The EOG records eye movements by taking advantage of the eye acting as a dipole. These channels are also labeled by the AASM shadowing the 10-20 system, as E1 (Left Eye) and E2 (Right Eye), and referenced to the opposing mastoid. By use of the dipole properties of the eye, the front of the retina is positively charged, and the back of the retina is negatively charged so, when a subject looks left, the front of their left eye would be closest to the E1 electrode and the recording for E1-M2 would show a downward (positive) deflection and the E2-M1 channel would show an upward (negative) deflection (Figure 47-1).

The final channel used to stage sleep is the chin EMG, which is recorded by referencing an electrode that is placed below the mandible to an electrode that is placed above the mandible. As the patient bites and clenches their jaw the muscle activity will result in "bursts" on the recorded chin channel (Figure 47-2).

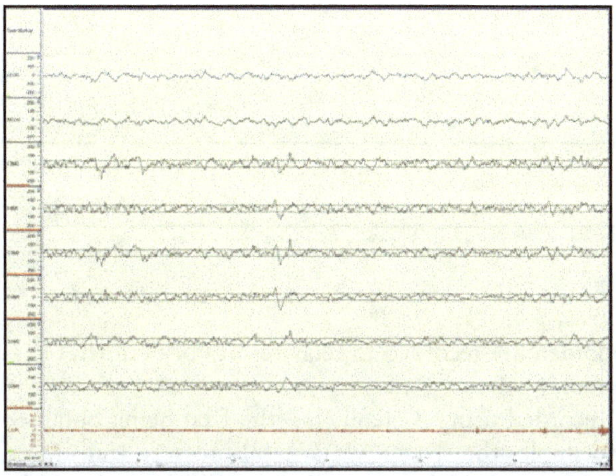

Figure 47-3. Sleep staging montage showing the EEG, EOG, and EMG channels.

Table 47-1

Characteristics of Each Sleep Stage

Wake (W): EEG consisting of alpha (8 to 12 Hz) activity emitted from the occipital area, along with high chin amplitude.
NREM Sleep
N1: The discontinuation of alpha. The EEG will contain low amplitude, mixed frequency EEG. The EOG will display slow rolling eye movements, and the chin will decrease in amplitude when compared with that of W. N2: Will contain EEG showing K-complexes and/or sleep spindles, dominant in the central EEG channels. K-complexes are sharp, quick negative wave forms that are tapered with a slower positive return. Sleep spindles are short bursts of activity that range from 11 to 16 Hz, and are 0.5 second in length or greater. N3: EEG consisting of Delta activity (0.5 to 2 Hz), at least 20% of the epoch, dominant in the frontal EEG channels.
REM Sleep
REM: The EEG will again contain low-amplitude, mixed-frequency EEG. Often, some EEG waves will appear like a "saw tooth." The EMG amplitude will be low, and the EOG will display sharp eye movement.

The combination of the EEG, EOG, and chin EMG is reviewed together for staging requirements and marked accordingly. Also marked, or scored, during the sleep staging are arousals, which are brief disruptions, greater than 3 seconds, in sleep indicated by an increase in the EEG frequency. A sleep staging montage is shown in Figure 47-3 and the characteristics of each sleep stage are noted in Table 47-1.

In addition to the recording and staging of sleep, respiratory channels are recorded. These channels are recorded to monitor the patient's inspiratory and expiratory airflow, and the expansion and

Figure 47-4. Montage of respiratory channels, including airflow, nasal pressure, end tidal carbon dioxide wave forms and respiratory inductance plethysmography channels, including ribcage and abdominal motion and their sum.

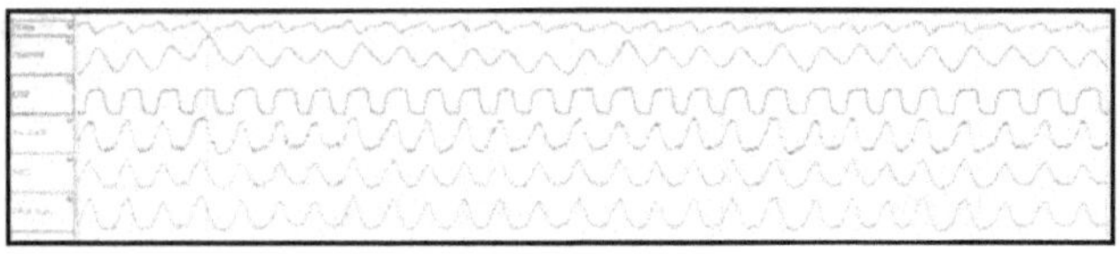

Figure 47-5. Bursts of snoring recorded with the snoring microphone.

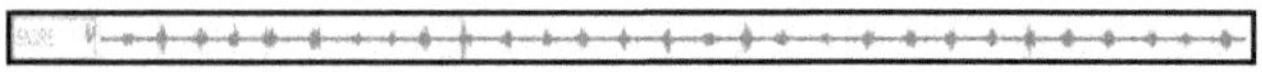

contraction movement of the thorax and abdomen are recorded to relay respiratory effort. These channels are critical to the detection of respiratory events.

Airflow of pediatric patients is typically recorded using 3 channels—the first being obtained by using an oral-nasal thermistor, or thermocouple, the second via a nasal pressure transducer, and the third by recording the capnogram, since end-tidal carbon dioxide ($ETCO_2$) should be recorded in this patient population to screen for hypoventilation. The oral-nasal thermistor is a small device that is placed below the patient's nose, and above their mouth. Typically there are small prongs that sense temperature difference that extend slightly in front of the nasal openings and another that extends in front of the mouth. Air exhaled from the patient will be warmer than the air inhaled, producing a waveform signal for this channel. A nasal pressure transducer is the most sensitive of the airflow devices and often the waveform is relied on heavily to detect some of the more subtle respiratory events. As the name indicates, it monitors pressure by means of a cannula, similar to that used to provide supplemental oxygen to a patient. This typically is the most difficult to place on a pediatric patient, and may require vigilance throughout the night to keep the patient from removing it. Lastly, the capnogram is essential in verifying $ETCO_2$ values, yet it is the least sensitive of the devices in relaying airflow disruption. Because of the way the capnogram signal is produced, the waveform can be delayed from one second to several seconds from those of the other airflow signals and, in some instances, the lesser respiratory events may not be as clearly distinguishable.

The expansion and contraction of the patient's thorax and abdomen are recorded using respiratory inductance plethysmography, which consists of elastic belts that have a wire embedded in them—almost in waveform pattern. An RIP belt is placed over the thorax area and another over the abdominal area, each creating a separately recorded qualitative signal. These 2 signals are also combined to create an additional channel termed *sum*. As the patient breathes, the thorax and abdomen expand or contract, and the belts along with them. There is a current passed through the waveform pattern wire in the belts—not through the patient—creating a magnetic field. This magnetic field changes as the distances in the waveform-patterned wire change, thereby producing a signal in the form of a waveform. Correct placement of the belts is important, as well as monitoring of the belts' correct location overnight during the PSG. During the review of the PSG, the quality of the signals should be taken into consideration, and it should also be understood that the belts detect movement, not effort. Figure 47-4 depicts the montage of respiratory channels recorded during PSG.

Adding to the list of recorded respiratory channels is the oxygen saturations (SpO_2), recorded via pulse oximetry, and a snore sensor. The snore sensor is a small device, typically ranging in the diameter size of a dime to a quarter, which is taped to the patient's neck, lateral to the larynx, to sense vibrations caused by snoring. The snore channel displays bursts of activity in the signal when snoring occurs (Figure 47-5).

These channels are then reviewed, at which point respiratory events are then scored by using AASM-established criteria (Table 47-2).

Table 47-2

Pediatric Respiratory Events: Simply Defined

Obstructive apnea: A period where airflow has stopped and effort to breathe is present throughout the event.
Central apnea: A period where airflow has stopped and effort to breathe is not present throughout the event.
Mixed apnea: A period where airflow has stopped and effort to breathe is partially present during the event.
Hypopnea: A period of reduced airflow with effort to breathe throughout the event.
Periodic breathing: A period of several—3 or more—central apneas together.
Note: Periodic breathing is a common occurrence in the younger pediatric population, especially during REM, but concern should be given if the events are associated with decreases in oxygen saturation (SpO_2), elevated $ETCO_2$, or it is showing unusual disruption to the sleep progression.
Hypoventilation: Where more than 25% of the patient's total sleep time shows an end tidal CO_2 value greater than 50 mm Hg.

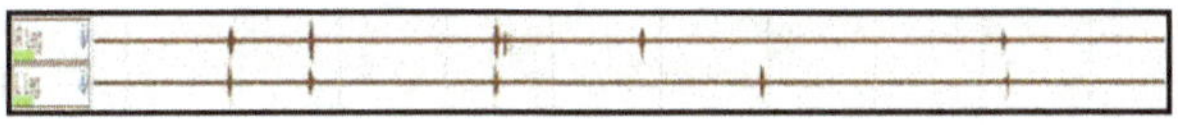

Figure 47-6. Bursts of muscle activity recorded with limb EMG.

A PSG will also include at least one ECG channel, derived from a modified ECG lead II and torso location. The ECG is reviewed during the scoring process, where arrhythmias will be scored and noted.

EMGs are not limited to being applied to just the chin, but also to the patient's leg. EMG electrodes are applied at the tibialis anterior location to detect limb movements. Some patients will have leg movements during sleep, in which case the leg EMG channels will display bursts of activity (Figure 47-6). If these movements happen frequently enough during sleep they will be scored as periodic limb movements of sleep.

The position of the patient should also be noted in the PSG recording, either by the recording technician's observations, or by a sensor that indicates the position as a channel in the PSG group of channel, called a montage. Audio and video are vital additions to the pediatric PSG, and can be useful to help determine what is taken place during certain times of the recording.

When all of these channels are combined in a single montage, the result is a powerful diagnostic tool that provides a wealth of information about the characteristics of sleep and breathing in a child over a prolonged period of time. Figures 47-7 and 47-8 show the full montage of PSG channels. By applying standard procedures in a child-friendly and in patient-focused environments, it is possible to get high quality, reproducible PSG studies on children of all ages and developmental stages.

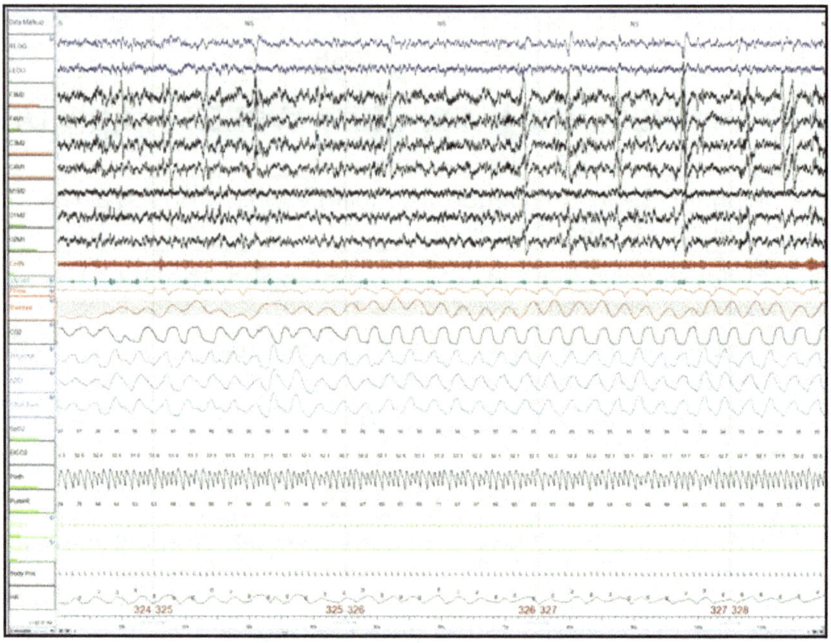

Figure 47-7. Full PSG montage showing regular breathing and snoring activity.

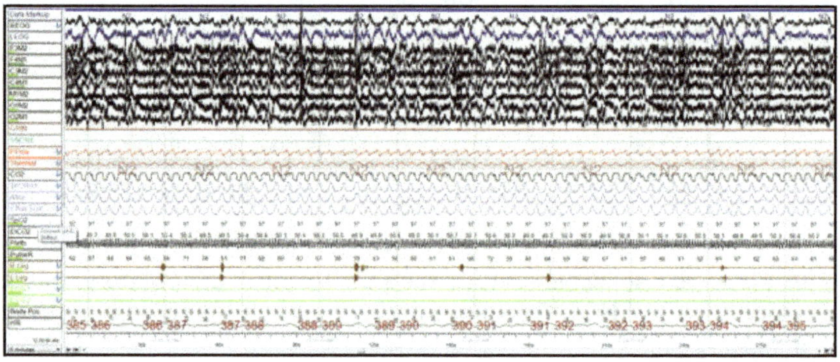

Figure 47-8. Full PSG montage showing bursts of limb activity consistent with periodic leg movements.

Suggested Readings

Aurora RN, Lamm CI, Zak RS, et al. Practice parameters for the non-respiratory indications for polysomnography and multiple sleep latency testing in children. *SLEEP.* 2012;35(11)1467-1473.

Aurora RN, Zak RS, Karippot A, et al. Practice parameter for the respiratory indications for polysomnography in children. *SLEEP.* 2011;34(3):379-388.

Beck SE, Marcus CL. Pediatric polysomnography. *Sleep Med Clin.* 2009;4(3):393-406.

Berry RB, Budhiraja R, Gottlieb DJ, et al. Rules for scoring respiratory events in sleep: update of the 2007 AASM Manual for the Scoring of Sleep and Associated Events. Deliberations of the Sleep Apnea Definitions Task force of the American Academy of Sleep Medicine. *J Clin Sleep Med.* 2012; 8(5):597-619.

QUESTION 48

Which of My Patients Should Have a Polysomnogram?

Aaron S. Chidekel, MD

Polysomnography (PSG) remains (and likely will remain) the gold standard for the diagnosis and management of pediatric sleep disorders. It can be performed for both respiratory and nonrespiratory indications (Table 48-1). However, it is a complex and labor intensive test that requires the child, along with a parent, to spend a night away from the home in a clinical testing environment. While PSG testing can be performed on infants and children of all ages and developmental abilities, a certain amount of tolerance and cooperation is required. Rarely, some patients (or parents) will not be able to tolerate the study procedures or environment, but this is very uncommon. Obtaining the PSG study in a center with pediatric experience and expertise will further increase the likelihood of a successful and atraumatic testing experience that obtains high quality and interpretable results. It is recommended that referring pediatric practitioners familiarize themselves with the experience and comfort levels of their local sleep laboratory with pediatric PSG. Obviously, those physicians in proximity to a children's hospital with an accredited pediatric sleep laboratory are able to refer to a sleep laboratory that exclusively tests infants and children. Referring physicians should familiarize themselves with the local referral practices as well. Some sleep programs will allow for direct referral of patients to the sleep laboratory for testing, whereas others require evaluation by a sleep medicine specialist prior to allowing the test to proceed. Other sleep medicine programs will allow direct referral by certain physicians and not others; and still other sleep programs will allow direct referral of certain groups of patients to the sleep laboratory while others must be seen by a sleep medicine specialist prior to testing.

In childhood, PSG testing is most frequently ordered for respiratory indications. As childhood obstructive sleep apnea syndrome is a common condition and the frequency of snoring in children is high, the most common clinical reason for obtaining a PSG is to evaluate a symptomatic child for OSA. PSG is highly sensitive and specific and is the definitive test for this diagnosis. Children with some combination of snoring, mouth breathing, daytime sleepiness or behavior changes, enlarged tonsils and/or adenoids, nasal congestion, and restless, disrupted sleep are all candidates for PSG to diagnose and treat OSA. Patients requiring positive airway pressure therapy to treat OSA will require PSG for titration of this therapy as well. Children who remain symptomatic

Chidekel AS, ed. *Curbside Consultation in Pediatric Sleep Disorders: 49 Clinical Questions* (pp. 221-223)

Table 48-1

Common Indications for Polysomnography Testing

Respiratory Indications
• Diagnosis and management of obstructive sleep apnea syndrome • Positive airway pressure titration • Evaluation of sleep-related hypoventilation • In select cases of apparent life-threatening events • Management of children with chronic respiratory failure and technology dependence
Nonrespiratory Indications
• Suspected periodic limb movement disorder • In combination with multiple sleep latency testing to evaluate for narcolepsy • Complex parasomnias • To assist in the diagnosis of restless legs syndrome

for about 6 to 8 weeks after adenotonsillectomy or who had severe OSA prior to surgery will also require a follow-up PSG. Infants with apparent life-threatening events and infants and children in whom there is suspicion for central apnea or hypoventilation will require PSG testing (including measurement of end tidal carbon dioxide levels) as well.

Less frequently, PSG will be indicated in the evaluation of nonrespiratory sleep disorders in childhood. For example, PSG is rarely, if ever, indicated in the evaluation of routine parasomnias, such as straightforward nightmares and/or night terrors, as the clinical history is sufficiently sensitive and specific. However, when parasomnias are complex, PSG can be useful to ensure that a less common condition, such as nocturnal epilepsy, is not present. Similarly, as sleep apnea can worsen parasomnias, any associated nocturnal respiratory symptoms should be assessed as well. In cases of complex parasomnias or other complex movements or behaviors during sleep, ensuring a good video recording during the PSG is important as is the documentation of any observations by the polysomnographic technician recording the study. The sleep-staging EEG will confirm in which stage of sleep any episodes are occurring, if they are indeed occurring during sleep. PSG can confirm the presence of periodic limb movements and is important in the diagnosis of periodic limb movement disorder; however, the diagnosis of restless legs syndrome is primarily based on clinical history. Children with true excessive daytime sleepiness will also require PSG testing accompanied by multiple sleep latency testing (MSLT). The MSLT, described in detail in Question 49, is performed the day following the overnight PSG study and formally quantifies daytime sleepiness and evaluates for sleep onset rapid eye movement periods that are seen in patients with narcolepsy.

Children with a multitude and variety of underlying conditions that can impact sleep and breathing are also candidates for PSG testing. Many of these conditions have been introduced elsewhere in this book. Common examples of children in whom regular PSG testing is often indicated and important are listed in Table 48-2. Children with chronic lung disease and those who are ventilator-dependent often require PSG to titrate therapy, and PSG is usually performed prior to the discontinuation of mechanical ventilatory support and tracheostomy tube decannulation. Children with cerebral palsy and other myopathies are also candidates for PSG testing. Children

Table 48-2

Examples of Common Underlying Conditions That May Require Polysomnography

- Trisomy 21
- Achondroplasia
- Prader-Willi syndrome
- Cerebral palsy
- Congenital myopathies and muscular dystrophies
- Craniofacial syndromes
- Sickle cell disease
- Selected cases of underlying respiratory disorders when a sleep disorder is suspected

with pediatric conditions, such as asthma, sickle cell disease, bronchopulmonary dysplasia cystic fibrosis, and pulmonary hypertension, are at higher risk of gas exchange abnormalities during sleep and/or obstructive sleep apnea syndrome; however, routine PSG testing is not generally recommended unless there are symptoms of a sleep disorder.

Summary

PSG testing is an incredibly valuable tool in the evaluation and management of a variety of daytime and nighttime pediatric signs and symptoms and underlying disorders when there is the indication to screen for, or where there are symptoms of, a respiratory or nonrespiratory sleep disorder. A number of children will require repeat testing. The complexity and labor-intensive nature of PSG testing should not detract from its appropriate clinical use. Pediatric PSG, ideally, should be performed in a sleep laboratory that has experience and interest in managing pediatric patients who can be challenging.

Suggested Readings

Aurora RN, Zak RS, Karippot A, et al. Practice parameters for the respiratory indications for polysomnography in children. *SLEEP.* 2011;34(3):379-388.

Aurora RN, Lamm CI, Zak RS, et al. Practice parameters for the non-respiratory indications for polysomnography and multiple sleep latency testing in children. *SLEEP.* 2012;35(11)1467-1473.

Beck SE, Marcus CL. Pediatric polysomnography. *Sleep Med Clin.* 2009 September;4(3):393-406.

Kotagal S, Nichols CD, Grigg-Damberger MM, et al. Non-respiratory indications for polysomnography and related procedures in children: an evidence-based review. *SLEEP.* 2012;35(11):1451-1466.

QUESTION 49

What Other Tests Are Used to Diagnose Sleep Disorders?

Todd Burchard, BS, RPSGT, RST and Aaron S. Chidekel, MD

Multiple Sleep Latency Test

A Multiple Sleep Latency Test (MSLT) comprises a series of naps that take place during the day and that are used to objectively measure a patient's sleepiness. The MSLT must be performed following a full overnight polysomnogram (PSG).

Indications

Typically, an MSLT is ordered for patients who have a suspected diagnosis of narcolepsy. History of excessive daytime sleepiness, cataplexy, and recurrent hypersomnia are all indications that would lead to an MSLT.

How Is a Multiple Sleep Latency Test Performed?

The overnight PSG should contain a minimum of 6 hours of sleep. Whereas the standards of MSLTs have been well defined for adults, standards for pediatrics have been rather difficult to determine. These values, such as 6 hours minimum of sleep, should be reviewed, perhaps on an individual patient basis, taking into consideration the patient's age and other factors that would determine if the patient would require more than 6 hours of sleep. The PSG should be free from other significantly sleep-fragmenting events, such as obstructive sleep apnea (OSA) and periodic limb movements of sleep. A PSG that indicates OSA would typically not be followed by an MSLT since the patient's sleepiness could be a result of disrupted sleep caused by the respiratory events. The OSA should be addressed and resolved first before further investigation into the patient's sleepiness is pursued.

Sleep logs, or sleep diaries, should be completed by the patient, preferably containing at least 2 weeks of recorded sleep history directly prior to the PSG and MSLT. Sleep logs are a simple

Chidekel AS, ed. *Curbside Consultation in Pediatric Sleep Disorders: 49 Clinical Questions* (pp. 225-229)

form that the patient or guardian completes, documenting the times the patient was asleep or awake. In circumstances in which the parent is completing the logs, one must take into consideration that the logs are documenting the parent's observations, and periods of wake or sleep may be missed. Also, in cases where the patient is completing the logs, there could be a fear to self-report long periods of wake during the night, or naps during the day.

MSLT naps are 4 to 5 nap "opportunities" that occur at 2-hour intervals through the day, with the first nap beginning 1.5 to 3 hours after "lights on" of the PSG. So, if the patient wakes up at 6:00 a.m., the first MSLT nap would start anywhere from 7:30 a.m. to 9:00 a.m. If the first nap starts at 7:30, the second would be at 9:30 a.m. If the first nap starts at 9:00 a.m., the second would be at 11:00 a.m.

It is extremely important that the patient is awake between naps. If the patient falls asleep between the MSLT naps, this could cause a reduced sleep drive, resulting in an inconclusive MSLT. The testing room will be bright and conducive to wakefulness after the PSG and between MSLT naps. This could involve having the patient get out of bed and take a walk, or sit upright in a chair and play a game with the parent until the next nap is to start. The patient should also avoid stimulating substances, such as chocolate or caffeine, and they should avoid strenuous activity, such as running. The day technologist will introduce themselves to the parent and patient well before the MSLT begins to provide the instructions of the test and to establish a partnership with the parent to ensure the patient is awake between nap times.

Before each nap, the patient and parent will be asked to mute their cell phones during nap times to avoid disrupted testing. The patient will be asked to "try to sleep" when the nap begins, or be asked to "allow yourself to fall asleep," and be told "if you can't sleep, rest quietly." Sometimes patients have anxiety believing that if they do not fall asleep that they ruin the test. The patient and parent will be reassured that they just need to try.

Any medications that the patient takes will be documented and taken into consideration since some medications can cause sleepiness. Also, just before the lights are shut off at each nap, the patient will be asked how sleepy he or she is, based on a scale. This answer is documented by the recording technologist to give the interpreting physician further clues as to the patient's perception of their own sleepiness.

During each nap, the patient is given 20 minutes from "lights off" to fall asleep—20 minutes being the amount of time it is thought to take a normal rested person to fall asleep. If the patient does not fall asleep in those 20 minutes, the nap is concluded. If, however, the patient does fall asleep during those 20 minutes, the test ends 15 minutes after the time they fall asleep, which is called sleep onset. So, if the patient falls asleep immediately at lights off, the test ends after 15 minutes. If the patient falls asleep 19.5 minutes into the nap, the test will end 15 minutes later, equaling 34.5 minutes. The amount of time from lights off to the first page, or epoch, of sleep is termed *sleep latency*.

In each MSLT nap, the left and right electrooculography channels, the electroenchephalography channels, chin electromyography, and ECG channels are recorded (Figure 49-1). Additional channels may be added at the discretion of the medical director.

What is abnormal

Once the MSLT naps are completed at the end of the day, the records are marked for stages of sleep, staged, and a report is generated (Figure 49-2). The report usually contains a graph that shows the stages of sleep observed. There will also be information regarding each nap, such as the time the nap started and ended, the amount of time it took to fall asleep (sleep latency), the amount of sleep (total sleep time), and if rapid eye movement (REM) was present. The sleep latency will

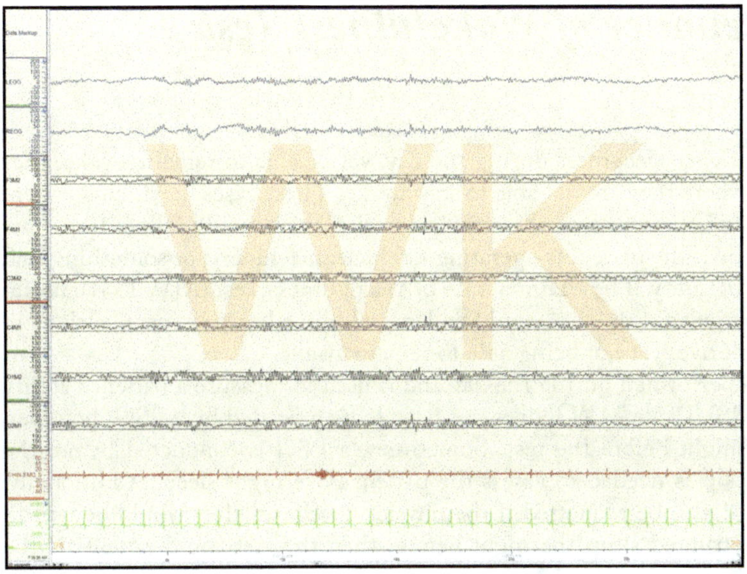

Figure 49-1. Typical montage for MSLT.

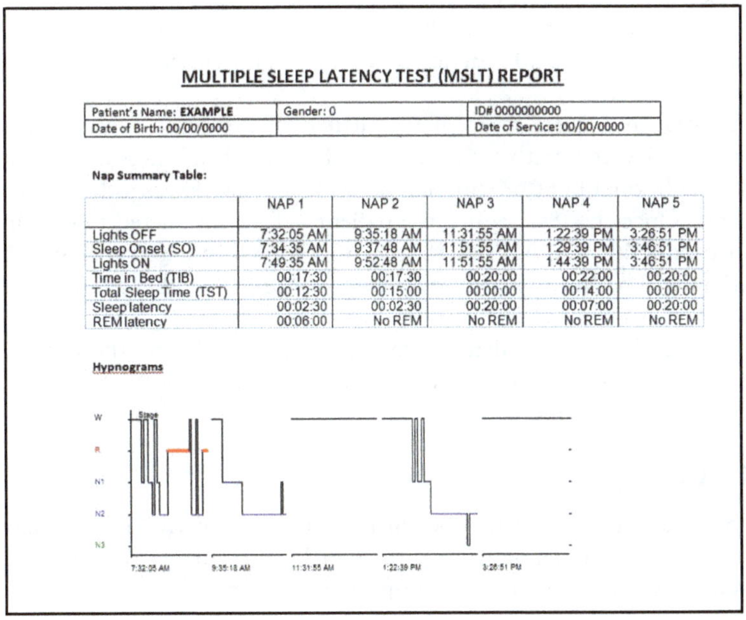

MULTIPLE SLEEP LATENCY TEST (MSLT) REPORT

Patient's Name: **EXAMPLE**	Gender: 0	ID# 0000000000
Date of Birth: 00/00/0000		Date of Service: 00/00/0000

Nap Summary Table:

	NAP 1	NAP 2	NAP 3	NAP 4	NAP 5
Lights OFF	7:32:05 AM	9:35:18 AM	11:31:55 AM	1:22:39 PM	3:26:51 PM
Sleep Onset (SO)	7:34:35 AM	9:37:48 AM	11:51:55 AM	1:29:39 PM	3:46:51 PM
Lights ON	7:49:35 AM	9:52:48 AM	11:51:55 AM	1:44:39 PM	3:46:51 PM
Time in Bed (TIB)	00:17:30	00:17:30	00:20:00	00:22:00	00:20:00
Total Sleep Time (TST)	00:12:30	00:15:00	00:00:00	00:14:00	00:00:00
Sleep latency	00:02:30	00:02:30	00:20:00	00:07:00	00:20:00
REM latency	00:06:00	No REM	No REM	No REM	No REM

Hypnograms

Figure 49-2. Example of an MSLT report: In this case, the patient underwent 5 nap trials and had a mean sleep latency of 10:24 minutes, which is normal. One SOREMP was noted in the first nap.

then be averaged. If the average sleep latency of the MSLT is equal to or less than 8 minutes, and REM is observed in 2 or more of the naps, termed *sleep onset REM periods* (SOREMPs), then the patient would be considered positive for narcolepsy. A sleep latency of less than 8 minutes without SOREMPs is consistent with excessive sleepiness or hypersomnia.

Maintenance of Wakefulness Test

Indications

Although people may experience sleepiness during the day, yet be able to remain awake, they may also experience episodes where they are not able to stay awake. These cases in which a patient is unable to remain awake—or believes he or she remains awake, yet actually falls asleep—are extremely concerning, especially if the patient is operating a vehicle, machinery, or something that requires alertness for the sake of safety. The Maintenance of Wakefulness Test (MWT) is a useful tool in situations where the patient's sleepiness would endanger him or her, or others, such as in cases of a teenager wanting to drive, yet not being able to remain awake.

The MWT is a test that is performed during the day and is used to measure a patient's ability to remain awake. Unlike an MSLT, the MWT does not have to be preceded by a PSG; however, adequate sleep is needed the night before the test. Sometimes, a PSG is conducted before the MWT if the clinician believes it is needed to assess the patient's overnight sleep. Additionally, sleep logs, or sleep diaries, will also be requested if the physician believes they would be useful. If the patient experiences interrupted sleep the night before, then the test could potentially be rescheduled.

The MWT is a series of 4 assessments that occur at 2-hour intervals through the day, with the first assessments starting 1.5 to 3 hours after the patient has awakened from his or her overnight sleep. Each assessment is scheduled to last up to 40 minutes. If the patient falls asleep during those 40 minutes, that assessment is concluded.

The patient performs the MWT in a quiet room, while sitting in a chair in a recumbent position, or on a bed with the head elevated, with a single light (about the brightness of a night light) on behind the patient. No additional light or stimulation, such as television or other noise, is allowed during the assessments. Once the test begins, the patient will be instructed to remain awake by the sleep technician conducting the MWT. If sleep is recorded, the technician will awaken the patient and the patient will be free to watch television and turn the lights on until the next scheduled assessment.

The channels recorded during the MWT are identical to those recorded during the MSLT, right and left EOG channels, EEG channels (F4-M1, F3-M2, C4-M1, C3-M2, O2-M1, O1-M2), chin EMG, and ECG or EKG channels.

What Is Abnormal?

Ideally, the patient should be able to remain awake the entire 40 minutes of all 4 assessments of the MWT. When a patient is unable to remain awake through a MWT, further steps will be explored by the physician. In some cases, a stimulant or wake-promoting medication is prescribed.

Actigraphy

An actigraph is typically a watch-like device that the patient wears for a certain amount of time that records movement in order to relay activity. The time periods with recorded activity (motion) are interpreted as periods of wake, as opposed to periods of little to no activity being interpreted as sleep.

Actigraphy can be used with sleep logs, or sleep diaries, to further investigate the patient's wake and sleep times.

Sleep Apps for Smart Phones

There is currently an explosion in "sleep apps," designed for popular cell phones and other digital devices. Applications (apps) designed to help people fall asleep, awaken at the appropriate time and from the appropriate stage of sleep, and to simply keep track of their sleep habits are available. Some of these apps have content and tools to treat insomnia and some are simply digital sleep logs. None of these apps are approved by the Food and Drug Administration as a true medical device and, therefore, they cannot be recommended to diagnose or treat any sleep disorder. Obviously, the efficacy or even real-world effectiveness or impact of any of these products on sleep and health is unknown.

Suggested Readings

Aran A, Einen M, Lin L, Plazzi G, Nishino S, Mignot E. Clinical and therapeutic aspects of childhood narcolepsy-cataplexy: a retrospective review study of 51 children. *SLEEP* 2010;33(10):1457-1464.

Aurora RN, Lamm CI, Zak RS, et al. Practice parameters for the non-respiratory indications for polysomnography and multiple sleep latency testing for children. *SLEEP* 2012;35(11):1467-1473.

Morgenthaler T, Alessi C, Friedman L, et al. Practice parameters for the use of actigraphy in the assessment of sleep and sleep disorders: an update for 2007. *SLEEP* 2007;30(4):519-529.

Standards of Practice Committee of the American Academy of Sleep Medicine. Practice parameters for clinical use of the multiple sleep latency test and the maintenance of wakefulness test. *SLEEP* 2005;28(1):113-121.

FINANCIAL DISCLOSURES

Dr. Louella Amos has no financial or proprietary interest in the materials presented herein.

Dr. Kari Baber has no financial or proprietary interest in the materials presented herein.

Dr. Suzanne E. Beck has no financial or proprietary interest in the materials presented herein.

Dr. Anita Bhandari has not disclosed any relevant financial relationships.

Dr. Michael Blechner has no financial or proprietary interest in the materials presented herein.

Todd Burchard has no financial or proprietary interest in the materials presented herein.

Dr. Christina Calamaro has no financial or proprietary interest in the materials presented herein.

Dr. Johanna Carpenter has not disclosed any relevant financial relationships.

Dr. Mohammad Cheema has no financial or proprietary interest in the materials presented herein.

Dr. Aaron S. Chidekel has no financial or proprietary interest in the materials presented herein.

Dr. Jennifer L. Curran has no financial or proprietary interest in the materials presented herein.

Dr. Lynn A. D'Andrea has no financial or proprietary interest in the materials presented herein.

Dr. Carl Gartner has no financial or proprietary interest in the materials presented herein.

Dr. Ritu Grewal has no financial or proprietary interest in the materials presented herein.

Dr. Robert Heinle has not disclosed any relevant financial relationships.

Dr. Cheyenne Hughes-Reid has no financial or proprietary interest in the materials presented herein.

Dr. Persephone Jones has no financial or proprietary interest in the materials presented herein.

Dr. Lewis J. Kass has no financial or proprietary interest in the materials presented herein.

Dr. Holger Link has no financial or proprietary interest in the materials presented herein.

Dr. Floyd Livingston has no financial or proprietary interest in the materials presented herein.

Dr. Jennifer L. Maher has not disclosed any relevant financial relationships.

Jennifer A. Marriner has no financial or proprietary interest in the materials presented herein.

Dr. Meghan McAuliffe Lines has not disclosed any relevant financial relationships.

Dr. Raj Padman has no financial or proprietary interest in the materials presented herein.

Dr. Vandna Passi has not disclosed any relevant financial relationships.

Dr. David A. Paul has no financial or proprietary interest in the materials presented herein.

Dr. Amy Renwick has not disclosed any relevant financial relationships.

Dr. Marianne C. San Antonio has no financial or proprietary interest in the materials presented herein.

Dr. Vanessa Shanks has not disclosed any relevant financial relationships.

Dr. Ambika Shenoy has not disclosed any relevant financial relationships.

Dr. Jennifer Shroff Pendley has not disclosed any relevant financial relationships.

Dr. Gabor Szuhay has no financial or proprietary interest in the materials presented herein.

Dr. Ignacio E. Tapia has not disclosed any relevant financial relationships.

Dr. Rhonda Walter has not disclosed any relevant financial relationships.

Dr. Rocio Zeballos-Chavez has no financial or proprietary interest in the materials presented herein.

INDEX

For Product Safety Concerns and Information please contact our EU representative GPSR@taylorandfrancis.com
Taylor & Francis Verlag GmbH, Kaufingerstraße 24, 80331 München, Germany

www.ingramcontent.com/pod-product-compliance
Lightning Source LLC
LaVergne TN
LVHW080650011026
849160LV00014B/1372

* 9 7 8 1 6 1 7 1 1 6 0 1 8 *